Menopause and Me

....

Embracing the Change, Celebrating Womanhood, Wellness Strategies for African American Women in Menopause.

Empowering Black Women!

•

TARA M. IVERSEN

....

Copyright © 2021 Tara M. Iversen

All rights reserved.

CONTENTS

INTRODUCTION 7

CHAPTER 1: UNDERSTANDING MENOPAUSE 11

    BLACK WOMANHOOD 11

    I CAN FEEL IT COMING 17

    THE SCIENCE BEHIND MENOPAUSE 21

CHAPTER 2: WHAT DOES BEING MENOPAUSAL FEEL LIKE? 25

    THINNING HAIR 26

    DRY AND LOOSER SKIN 29

    WEIGHT GAIN AND CHANGING BODY SHAPE 31

    LIBIDO CHANGES 33

    ACHES, PAINS, AND HOT FLASHES 35

    NO MORE PERIODS 37

    MENTAL HEALTH ISSUES 38

CHAPTER 3: ALTERNATIVE AND NATURAL TREATMENT ... 43

    FOR STRONGER AND NOURISHED HAIR AND NAILS 45

    FOR GLOWING AND SUPPLE SKIN 46

    FOR WEIGHT-LOSS AND BODY SCULPTING 49

    FOR INCREASED SEX DRIVE 51

    FOR PHYSICAL DISCOMFORT 54

    FOR A HEALTHY MIND, BODY, AND SOUL 55

    EXERCISE 56

    YOGA 57

- Breathing Exercises and Meditation 58
- Cognitive Behavioral Therapy 60
- Hypnotherapy 62
- Massage Therapy and Aromatherapy 63
- Food and Drink 64

CHAPTER 4: PROFESSIONAL SUPPORT AND TRADITIONAL TREATMENT 67

- When To Seek Professional Support 67
- Trusting Your Doctor 68
- Preparing For an Appointment 70
- Hormone Replacement Therapy 73
- Types of HRT 74
- Other Prescribed Treatments 75

CHAPTER 5: LIVING YOUR BEST LIFE WITH MENOPAUSE .. 77

- An Inspiring Morning Routine 77
- Support At Work 80
- A Colorful Social Life 82
- A Calming Nighttime Routine 86
- Going On Vacation 90

CHAPTER 6: FAMILY, RELATIONSHIPS, AND THE MENOPAUSAL WOMAN 93

- Family 93
- Older Generations 94
- Teenaged Children 95
- Alone Time 97
- Friends 99
- Romantic Relationships 102

CHAPTER 7: MENOPAUSE AND BEYOND 107

    STAY IN TOUCH WITH YOUR DOCTOR 108

    MAINTAIN HOLISTIC HEALTH 112

    PASS IT ON 116

    ENJOY YOUR LIFE 117

CONCLUSION 121

REFERENCES 125

Introduction

Menopause. It shouldn't be a dirty word, especially as virtually half of the population will go through it at some point in their lives, but sometimes it feels like it is, with society brushing it under the carpet like a taboo subject. It is a part of womanhood we can't avoid, so it's about time we talk about it, embrace it, and be honest with ourselves and others about our unique journeys. Not only will sharing and discussing our concerns, questions, and laughable moment, help our fellow menopausal sisters learn and relate, but younger women will feel guided and prepared for what is yet to come. By opening the conversation, we will begin to understand this phenomenon in more depth and discover that we aren't alone in our struggles which will also help us all feel more empowered and confident enough to continue to live a 'normal' and fruitful life, in spite of menopause.

I'm April; a mother of a wonderful adult daughter and grandmother of two. For the past four years I have been going through menopause, doing my best to navigate around my symptoms, worries, and evolving identity as a Black woman. I understand, through first-hand experience, that many African American women feel ashamed or silenced by this change because we are not only faced with being of a certain age that isn't always represented positively, but we are also challenged by racial stigmas and prejudice as well as being female in a patriarchal world.

But fear not! Although all of our experiences will be different, I know that the words of wisdom I am going to share with you will help you feel more comfortable with the journey you are about to embark on—or are on at the moment. This book will also guide you in a way that will make you more knowledgeable and arm you with the tools you need to make it to the light at the end of, what can sometimes feel like, a dark menopausal tunnel. I will offer balanced, honest, and compassionate insight with personal anecdotes, recommendations, and treatments that I am sure will resonate with you and be beneficial to you at some stage of your journey.

I am passionate about sharing this information as widely as possible because I want my grandchildren to grow up in a world that understands that menopause is normal, natural, and something that women shouldn't be afraid of any more. I have seen how this challenging time has affected my friends and family, directly and indirectly, physically and emotionally, so I think this is the only way to stop the stigma and put a pause on menopausal shame.

When managed well, menopause does not spell the end of womanhood, sexuality, or mental wellness, but it can be the start of an enlightening new chapter and together we can make it as smooth-sailing as possible. So, I encourage you to be bold, brave, and open-minded and continue reading to learn more about your evolving, thriving, and beautiful body.

Chapter 1:
Understanding Menopause

The female experience of menopause is by no means monolithic but there are of course some scientifically proven changes that occur in all of our bodies which definitively indicate that we are going through this rite of passage. Before we learn exactly what menopause is and understand how, and to what extent, this phenomenon affects us, it is important to know who we are before it kicks in. So, let's discuss what it means to be, not only a woman, but a Black woman in America today.

Black Womanhood

According to Catalyst research, in 2019 Black women made up just 12.9% of the American female population. When comparing this to the fact that 60% of females are white, it is clear that we are a minority and this comes with its challenges. Being a minority in the Western world often means that our voices are not heard and we are usually poorly represented when it comes to political decisions made about the way we live, work, and are treated in the healthcare system, for example. Because of this, although our individual lives may be full of achievement, strength, and positivity, our collective experience is often blighted with pain, injustice, and discrimination. Black women have faced historical dehumanization, oppression, and violence that has evolved into institutional and structural racism across the United States and beyond. We are sadly fetishized in the media, which leaves our #BlackGirlMagic feeling tarnished. We are presented as loud or un-educated, which silences and invalidates our voices, and we are told that we are the least desirable group on dating apps (Linshi 2014), wreaking havoc with our self-esteem.

Fortunately, with a strong sense of community and sisterhood among Black women, we are becoming increasingly vocal about the need for change and are rewriting our own definitions of Black womanhood and femininity. We openly and loudly empower and uplift our fellow sisters and are slowly regaining control of our narrative. With the resurgence of the Black Lives Matter movement forcing the world to listen to our concerns, demands, and realities and the increasing use of social media highlighting our talents as well as the inequalities we face, people of all races are also starting to tune in to our more positive, inclusive, and rounded representation of who we are, and this is a positive step in the right direction.

We are mothers. Black mothers are wise, doting, and tender but also fierce, bold, and resilient. We often make sacrifices in order to uplift, inspire, and guide the next generation with little to no recognition but we continue to do it out of love. Characters such as Aunt Viv in *The Fresh Prince of Bel-Air* and Claire Huxstable from *The Cosby Show* demonstrated these real-life qualities beautifully and are looked upon fondly by people of all ages and races. These mothers, although fictional, depicted our deep sense of duty to raise our children in positive environments and with ample opportunities, and showed that we make it our mission to work hard and set a good example for them. Being a mother often gives Black women a sense of purpose and fulfillment and many of us feel proud to carry this title and pass on generational wisdom to help the Black community not just survive, but thrive. Furthermore, with 30% of African American households being run by women, compared to just 9% of white homes (Mental Health America, 2020), many Black people grow up in multi-generational matriarchal households; being raised by Black women, who were raised by Black women, so it is little wonder we feel such a connection to motherhood.

Black women are successful and educated. We are an ambitious, talented, and forward-thinking group of people which is supported by the fact that, according to Essence Magazine, Black women have been consistently acquiring degrees at an increasingly high rate for the past eight years (Davis, 2020). What's more, one of the leading scientists who developed the

Covid-19 vaccine in 2020, was Kizzmekia Corbett, PhD—a Black woman, and the second woman to ever be Secretary of State is Condoleezza Rice—another Black woman. Our success isn't limited to science and politics; It spans across music, sports, business, entertainment and so much more, showing that our minds are truly brilliant!

Black women are leaders and activists. Kristina Button says in her 2021 blog, *In Our Mothers' Gardens,* that we are activists by default because the "racial hierarchy in America ensures that Black women must fight for themselves and everyone else". She believes that it is a quality that has been embedded in us because of generations of oppression.

To be an activist you need tenacity, a captivating personality, and eloquence and we have all of these qualities in abundance. It is ingrained into our being, whether we recognize it or not, which is why people like Michelle Obama, Viola Davis, and Oprah demand our attention with their presence and are popular among people from all walks of life. We aren't afraid to stand up for what we believe in, raise awareness, and shake up the world in the process as activist and Time magazine's Person of the Year 2017, Tarana Burke did. Burke founded the "Me Too" group that later evolved into the #MeToo movement which helped people stand in solidarity with others who have been victims of sexual assault; an international movement for justice. Black culture also leads the way with creativity, inspiring fashion, dance, and music, showing that we are truly innovative changemakers.

We are beautiful, desirable, and admired by many. Beauties such as Adut Akech, Winnie Harlow, and Precious Lee are making waves in the modeling industry and have paved the way for many aspiring young Black models. These women showcase our diverse beauty in the form of tight curls, unique skin and sexy curves and are in demand by some of the most high-profile brands, proving that Black can and should be considered beautiful. This industry unfortunately has a toxic history of exclusivity and diversity issues that are still prevalent today but seeing Black faces and bodies like these dominating catwalks and on covers of magazines is empowering and encouraging.

If we go back to times of slavery or even as recent as the 1960s civil rights movement, our bodies, hair, and features were ridiculed and paraded around to be inspected and judged. Black women were seen as ugly and masculine, and, because our features and skin tones were the farthest from the white male, we were also valued as virtually worthless. Fast-forward to today, and things are far from perfect or equal, but our shape, skin, and hair are even being emulated and admired, with Beyonce's *Brown Skin Girl* lyrics echoing satisfyingly in our ears: "Same skin that was broken, be the same thing takin' over" (Beyonce, 2019).

Black women are also human. We grow, we love, we cry, and we age. Crying and feeling weak is often looked at as a negative but it shouldn't be. It is impossible, not to mention unhealthy, to be positive and emotionless all the time, so although the "strong Black woman" trope can be empowering, it can also be damaging. It often makes us feel as though we need to cut off our own valid and raw emotions in order to be considered a 'real' black woman which can take its toll on our mental health. Over seven million Black people in the US have mental health issues, so it is important that this Black female strength is balanced with an allowance for vulnerability and free expression.

Aging is also human but, as we become older, it is easy for Black women to feel invisible in a world that values youth. Thankfully, there are groups out there that recognize that aging is dynamic and exciting and what was considered old 30 years ago, is now the prime of life. People are living longer, achieving more, and looking and feeling holistically healthier, so there's no reason why growing older shouldn't be celebrated.

In 2019, InStyle spoke to several Black women about aging and found that, although we do have some concerns when it comes to our mortality, growing older is a fact of life that our community actually isn't that bothered by. In fact, among the women they spoke to, most embraced looking and getting older and writer Kayla Greaves believes that this is due to our ancestry. In many traditional West African societies, elderhood was something to be admired and respected. It held great status and power which meant that appearing older could be beneficial. Even today, women like Angela Bassett and the late Cicely Tyson are known for aging gracefully with their graying hair and natural wrinkles being seen as beautiful. Black women tend to celebrate life and see aging as a way of indicating survival and accomplishment. So why do we feel more comfortable with this side of growing older than we do with the other changes that happen to our bodies?

I Can Feel It Coming

Our bodies are always changing. We lose our "baby fat", go through puberty and get taller over the years, evolving into adults and then we change some more. But when we get to a certain age, these changes can be a bit of a nuisance. The nuisance I am talking about at this time is the perimenopause. This is considered to be the transitional period before menopause which can be challenging, both physically and emotionally.

Perimenopause may begin as early as your mid-30s or as late

as your mid-50s. It can last years or just a short time but the main indication that you are going through it is having an unpredictable menstrual cycle. You may also experience heavier or lighter flows than usual, a sudden feeling of warmth that spreads across your body, also known as a "hot flash", sleep problems, and vaginal dryness. For some women, this turbulent time can affect their mood because of its instability and the fact that it is confirmation that you are heading towards a new chapter of life.

In the United States, the average girl starts her period at the age of 12. Before it comes, if we are fortunate enough, we learn about all the different types of sanitary products, best period practices and cycle expectations, and some parents even prepare "period parties" to celebrate their tween's upcoming coming-of-age milestone. When it finally comes, some feel excited to be entering into womanhood and despite the pain, we embrace it as something we have to go through as females.

As the months go by, our cycles usually become more regular and for the next 20–30 something years we spend approximately $6,360 on sanitary products (Bakar, 2020). Advertisements spend millions of dollars telling us that they can make our periods seemingly disappear through absorption, so that we can get on with our exciting and busy lives. Men are told not to ask about the 'P-word' so as not to come across as insensitive or rude and we try our hardest to pretend as though our period doesn't exist and yet, every month we go through the same feelings of moodiness, discomfort, and even pain. With the risk of sounding too graphic, that's an average of 1,215 ounces of blood, 3,360 days of cramps and 15,000 period products (Oerman, 2017), but like the strong women we are, we continue to power though; going to work, looking after the kids, and maintaining relationships while putting on weight, going gray, and feeling at our sexual peak.

Then one day, you are sitting at home, checking your emails and you realize that you are three days late with your period. You know for a fact that you aren't pregnant but you take a test anyway. Negative. A few days later, mother nature arrives (much to your relief) but it is twice as heavy and lasts four days longer than usual! Next month, you are three days late with barely any bleeding and the month after that it doesn't come at all. Then, just as you put on your Labor Day whites, guess who shows up six days earlier than expected.

Jokes aside, all of this perimenopausal inconsistency can be frustrating and even scary. What was once a predictable and manageable body has become unbalanced and erratic and this is not easy to deal with, as I learned about a year before my menopause. Perimenopause hit me hard but I was fortunate to only experience two of the classic symptoms; hot flashes and night sweats. They were unbearable and stopped me from having a peaceful night's sleep for months. The hot flashes made me feel as though I was on fire sometimes and I would sweat profusely, no matter where I was or what I was doing. I remember going shopping at a store and being hit with a sudden hot flash. I ran out to my car in desperate need of some AC and once I was inside, I had to take off my shirt and wipe away what felt like liters of sweat from my arms, chest, and stomach. Fortunately, I had tinted windows but this didn't hide the embarrassment and shame I felt afterwards. I decided not to return to the store that day because I didn't want anyone to see the sweat patches on my clothes, so I went home as a bit of a damp mess! Although not all of my vasomotor episodes (hot flashes and night sweats) were this bad, I know that they and other symptoms can be extremely distressing for some women. It is, however, an experience that almost all of us will go through at some point, so I hope that you don't feel isolated and are able to share your experiences with others to help lighten the load a little.

Of course, if at any point you feel as though your symptoms are too much to handle or you are unsure whether they are actually signs of perimenopause, please seek professional advice because they will be able to guide you and give any advice you need for your particular situation. Sometimes, the worry and anxiety surrounding the approach to menopause could be completely unnecessary as there are conditions such as hypothyroidism, hyperthyroidism, and even anxiety itself that can produce similar symptoms, so it's best to get checked out if you are at all apprehensive.

The Science Behind Menopause

It's the question you've been waiting for an answer to and that is, what is menopause? Although virtually all women go through it, the State of Menopause Study of 1,039 American women aged 40 to 65 stated that nearly a third of them (29%) never sought information about menopause before they experienced it and nearly half (45%) didn't know the difference between perimenopause and menopause itself (Gordon, 2021). So let's get into it.

Scientifically speaking, menopause is when someone's menstrual cycle and fertility comes to an end. It literally means the 'pause' (end) of your 'menses' (period). Doctors use two factors to confirm menopause has occurred and these are: when your ovaries stop producing estrogen and progesterone completely (hormones required for fertility) and when your period has not returned for 12 months or more. This usually means that it is something that is diagnosed after the fact. Women who are going through this 'waiting' time are often called menopausal or described as "going through menopause" and once they reach a full year with no periods or fertility hormones, they are considered post-menopausal. The process usually begins naturally around the age of 51 but it can start sooner and some surgeries or medical treatments can also trigger it, although the age at which it starts is mostly determined by your genes.

Women are born with a finite number of eggs in our ovaries. The ovaries not only produce these little potentials of life, but also release essential hormones that are needed to tell the body to menstruate, develop breasts, and grow hair in certain places. Each month during our menstrual cycle, an egg (or sometimes multiple eggs) is released and waits to be fertilized by sperm. If it is not, it is dispelled during our periods and this process repeats itself continuously, but as we age, our ovaries sense the emptying of our egg reserves and respond by slowing down the production of estrogen to reduce wastage. This shows just how intuitive our bodies are! In fact, by reducing estrogen levels, our bodies are also protecting us from age-related diseases such as breast, ovarian, and colorectal cancer because these are all estrogen dependent; using the hormone to grow and spread. This loss of fertility is also the body's way of protecting us from childbirth as carrying and delivering a baby becomes riskier with age. On average, a woman reaches her peak bone density at the age of 18, which is also when we are most fertile, whereas, during menopause our bone density tends to reduce, so carrying the weight of a baby at this age can come with more risks. Making a baby with older eggs can also have higher rates of chromosomal abnormalities, so the reduction of estrogen is no coincidence, just the beauty and wonder of our brilliant bodies protecting the next generation!

There are also several biomarkers that happen during menopause. These are chemical changes in our bodies that help doctors detect the onset menopause if you aren't entirely sure. One of the chemicals they will look for is dehydroepiandrosterone-sulfate, or thankfully just DHEAS. It is a molecule that is stored in the blood and is made from cholesterol. It is stored until it is needed to make sex hormones that maintain energy, muscle and bone health, and sexual function in both men and women but if low quantities are found in the body it can be an indicator of menopause. Ovarian testosterone will also decrease but testosterone will still remain in circulation as it is still produced by the adrenal glands.

Sex Hormone Binding Globulin (SHBG) levels actually increase as we grow older. SHBG is produced in the liver and is what binds the estrogen and testosterone together, helping them move around the body. When SHBG increases it can bind too many of these hormones and make them less effective in the body, resulting in menopausal symptoms.

Aging can also cause the formation of vitamin D to decrease. This vitamin is important because it is necessary for calcium absorption and calcium is one of the major structural components of bone. Because of its significant role in our bodies, vitamin D is usually one of the first levels checked and addressed by your doctor if they suspect that you are approaching menopause.

If you are someone who suffers from very painful or heavy periods or you have severe PMS symptoms, you may jump for joy at the idea of your body changing in this way and not having a period again, but unfortunately, managing menopause is not always as simple as saving money on sanitary products, taking vitamin supplements, and having chemical level and blood tests; these menopausal changes often have significant symptoms that can affect every aspect of our lives.

Chapter 2:
What Does Being Menopausal Feel Like?

With the reduction of hormones and varying levels of chemicals disrupting our natural balance, the run up to menopause is inevitably going to make our bodies change and feel different. These changes happen to women of all races, backgrounds, and nationalities but for Black women, some menopausal symptoms can be particularly difficult to face because of our unique identities, genetics, and upbringing. For example, an article on Endocrine Web states that Black and Latina women may begin perimenopause earlier, have a longer transition period to menopause, and experience more intense menopausal side effects. Study of Women's Health Across the Nation (SWAN) research also showed that Black women reach menopause two years earlier than the median age in the United States and professor Dr Nanette Santoro at the University of Colorado School of Medicine has said that this is probably due to our "lifestyle, socioeconomic status, and other stressors such as systemic racism and their long-term consequences" (Velez, 2014).

The way we view ourselves as individuals and as a community is important to us. As we've discussed, Black women often want to be seen as strong, beautiful and motherly leaders, so anything like menopausal symptoms that distort what we know to be our true reflections will be understandably challenging to deal with.

Thinning Hair

For all women, the way we wear our hair, its length, color, and texture often let people know a little bit about who we are and where we come from. In today's society it is also considered, right or wrong, an indicator of femininity. For example, the longer and more luscious your hair is, the more feminine you are considered. It is so linked to our public and personal identity that, for many women, a bad hair day is equal to a bad day, period, and this relationship between hair and self-esteem is evident throughout history, philosophy, and even religion.

From Marie Antoinette's outrageous wigs to the mohawks of 1970s punks, hair has been used to send out signals to others about our gender, class, status, age, marital status, group membership, and more. An interesting example of this would be the fact that ancient Egyptian queen, Cleopatra, would change her hairstyle to signal different things depending on where she was and who was around. She would wear it in a traditional Egyptian 'melon' style at home to de-emphasize her Greek roots and feel more accepted, but when traveling outside of Egypt, she would wear the hairstyles of a Greek queen; sectioned into curls and tied into a neat low bun, to celebrate her true cultural roots. This is very similar to cultural assimilation, which Black women are all too familiar with!

As well as this, from a young age, children are made aware of the value and desirability of an abundance of hair through the fictional stories we tell them. Fairytale characters such as Rapunzel, who would not have been rescued had it not been for her long and strong hair, have made many a young girl run around with stockings on her head, pretending she has the long flowing locks of this princess. In real life, this value is also reflected in that hair and beauty is a multibillion-dollar industry, with the average woman spending approximately $50,000 on her hair over her lifetime (Ellery, 2014). This is not just because we want to look good but also because society holds these strands in such high regard.

For Black women, our hair takes on even more of a role in our identity and is often described as our crown. The phrase "crowning glory" dates back to Biblical times and, according to 1 Corinthians 11:15, "but for a woman, if her hair is abundant, it is a glory to her; for her hair is given to her for a covering" (Ellery 2014). It even goes on to say that women who have an uncovered head are dishonorable "for she is on a level with her whose head is shaven" which adds a lot of pressure for us to maintain this 'crown' if we are of the Christian faith.

The heartfelt 2019 Oscar award-winning animation *Hair Love*, also showcased our particular affinity to our hair and it resonated with so many Black people across the world because of this. Our afros have been a symbol of activism, our locs are an indication of our spirituality, our cornrows were used as guidance and a technique to find freedom from slavery, and we often use hair styling and preening as a form of bonding with our fellow Black women. So when we go through menopause and our hair changes, it can feel like a low blow in many ways.

Sadly, one of the symptoms of going through menopause can be hair thinning. It can look less full as it sheds due to the reduction of estrogen; the hormone that promotes hair growth, density, and fullness. Some women will generally notice more hair brushing away as they style it and others may experience significant loss at the crown and at the sides of the head, known as female pattern hair loss (FPHL). But as India Arie's song *I Am Not My Hair* said, we should not feel defined by what we have or don't have on our heads, whether it be through choice or circumstance. We are still valuable and as fierce as Wakanda warriors, and, with the 2022 Oscars highlighting hair loss in a bizarre way, more and more people are recognizing and are more sympathetic toward any form of loss or thinning women go through. So, as much as this change may take some adjusting to, I urge you to maintain your confidence and sense of self-worth and beauty through it all.

Dry and Looser Skin

Our skin may also suffer as we go through menopause because our bodies stop producing as much collagen, with some studies showing that its production reduces by up to 30% in the first five years after menopause kicks in. Acne can also be a symptom. We may think that we have left our acne prone skin behind in our teen years, but if we see menopause for what it is, it's almost like going through another puberty, so the occurrence of pimples and spots is understandable.

We also tend to lose some fat under the skin and it loses its elasticity resulting in fine lines and wrinkles. This can be somewhat a concern to African American women in particular, as we worry if we will no longer fit into the "black don't crack" category! We are known for beautifully smooth complexions and vibrant tones; almost defying time and this youthful look has even helped ordinary women become known across the globe. For example, in January 2016 a Twitter photo of a mom and her twin daughters was retweeted more than 18,000 times and liked over 29,000 times (Booker, 2016) as people all over the world were left confused as to who was the mother out of the three beautiful women in the image.

High schooler Kaylan Mahomes added a caption that simply read "Mom, twin, and me" but the followers couldn't determine who was her twin and who was her mom because they all shared the same youthful glow. Many of the retweets of this post were accompanied by #blackdontcrack and the women were widely celebrated by people of all races, so when we are faced with the possibility of no longer being part of this celebration, it can feel a little disappointing.

Thankfully, skin care is a big part of the Black community as many of us have grown up moisturizing daily. No matter what part of the African diaspora we are in, we all have fond memories of our parents or family members dowsing us in coconut oil or shea butter before school, so we looked beautifully shiny, and carrying a spare tube of cocoa butter in our bags to treat ashy knees at the end of the day. But as we reach this time of life, we may find ourselves strangely becoming more sensitive to the creams we've used for years or find them not being as effective, so trying out new products may be necessary to maintain the complexion and moisturization we desire.

The higher levels of melanin in our skin also protects us from a lot of the sun's damaging rays, which is the biggest contributor to aging skin. As well as this, people with highly-melanated skin have a thicker dermis layer, which is the deeper layer of the skin that is full of collagen, so the aging process seems to take longer. We also produce more natural oils than fairer complexions and, while these can cause breakouts at times, when we age, they help keep the skin hydrated and prevent wrinkles.

Now, this doesn't mean that we are immune to aging, sun burn, or the effects of menopause completely, but it does give us a little bit of a leg up and we should continue to look after our skin in the best way we can.

Weight Gain and Changing Body Shape

Being menopausal is not directly associated with weight gain, but the fact that we are growing older and that our lifestyles generally become more sedentary is more likely to be the reason why we add on a few more pounds around this time. The fact that our muscle mass decreases with age is also why many of us put on weight when menopausal, because having less muscle tissue slows down the rate at which our bodies use calories i.e., our metabolism slows down. The increase of cortisol—the "stress hormone"—can also play a role in weight gain as it has been associated with fat accumulation, so as you get more stressed about the other menopause symptoms, its production increases and you gain weight. You then get stressed about the weight gain and this vicious circle continues, so try your best to relax and worry about as little as possible!

I know this is far easier said than done, but gaining weight can be very problematic, especially within African American society, as it can increase the risk of heart disease, diabetes, and high blood pressure, which are diseases that are already prevalent in our community. According to the National Institutes of Health, Black adults in the United States are nearly twice as likely to have type two diabetes than white adults and this racial disparity has been rising over the last 30 years (Hicklin, 2018), so if we add menopausal weight gain to this it can lead to some shocking and discouraging outcomes.

Although menopause on its own does not make you gain a significant amount of weight, it does, however, seem to have some impact on our body composition and fat distribution (Fenton, 2021). Studies show that women who are perimenopausal have increased fat on their abdomen, regardless of their age, so it is common for women to go from a pear shape, having a slimmer upper-body and wider hips, to more of an apple shape—a rounder mid-section. This is because, without enough estrogen, the body seems to selectively accumulate subcutaneous—below the skin—fat in the intra-abdominal compartment of the body and this shape has even earned itself a special name: 'menopot'.

Changes in the breasts can also occur during menopausal years. Loss of fullness, altering shape and size, unpredictable tenderness and aches, and even lumps can all make your breast feel different from how they did 10 years ago. These changes make it even more important to know what is normal for you so that you can seek help if or when something feels different and rule out anything more sinister than hormonal changes. The shape and size of your breasts changes because your lower levels of estrogen shut down your milk system and the glandular tissue in your breasts shrinks, making your breasts look less dense and fatty. Lumps occur if you have cysts that grow larger because of hormones. These are not cancerous and many women of all ages have them, even before menopause kicks in, so if they are normal for you, there is usually nothing to worry about.

The additional fat around the torso and buttocks may not seem like a problem in a society that values and praises 'thick' bodies now, but it is something to keep an eye on. After all, as long as you are healthy and happy, that's all that matters!

Libido Changes

Some women notice that their libido, or sex drive, changes during and post-menopause. Some may experience an increase, while others find that they have little to no interest in sexual intimacy at all. An increase in desire could be due to our minds being less preoccupied or worried about falling pregnant or being on our periods and a reduction in libido is often again down to our hormones; the lower testosterone and estrogen levels make it more difficult to feel aroused and we feel less sensitive to touching and stroking. This is generally normal and gradually occurs in both men and women as we age, but women are two to three times more likely to be affected (Menopause Health Centre Guide, 2022).

Not only are our minds affected in this way but menopause can also physically change our bodies in ways that make penetrative sexual intercourse painful. For example, it can cause vaginal dryness and tightness, because of a drop in blood supply to the vagina. You may also start to feel more tired, experience night sweats, and gain weight which some women will feel self-conscious about, making them not want to engage in anything as intimate as sex with someone else.

For many women, not having any sexual desire does not have a large impact on their overall sexuality or quality of life but it can be noticeable and challenging for their partners and threaten to weaken romantic relationships if not discussed openly and honestly. There is no 'normal' libido as everyone's sex drive is different but if the change becomes a concern for your relationship, it's a good idea to seek help.

On the other hand, if you are someone who used to enjoy sex, you may find this gradual decline in sexual desire to be a source of personal distress and lead to a sense of dissatisfaction. You may start to compare your sex life to other women who are not having this struggle and begin to feel as though there is something wrong with you. If we take this a little deeper, for Black women this can be particularly challenging because during slavery and the civil rights movements, we weren't allowed or given the opportunity to explore our sexuality or consent to sexual contact, so we now have an innate desire to reclaim our bodies in this way and menopause can feel as if we are being robbed of this.

The desire for sex, in its most primal form, is also the body's natural way to encourage the production of babies, so if we no longer have this desire, it can be a stark reminder that we are coming to the end of our maternal years. This can be difficult, daunting, and depressing for some to face, especially if you want to have children and haven't done so yet. But remember, being a biological mother does not define you as a woman and your value doesn't decrease as you pass child bearing years, whether you want children or not.

Aches, Pains, and Hot Flashes

Changes in the production of estrogen can affect the joints and the connective tissue that holds your bones together. Lack of this hormone increases inflammation which results in aches and pains, so these feelings are very common during menopause, with 60% of women in a study of 8,000 having increased muscle and joint discomfort (Elgaddal, 2021). Women over 50 are also more likely to develop things like osteoarthritis caused by wear and tear, and rheumatoid arthritis, which is an autoimmune disease that mistakenly attacks the cells that line your joints. Both can be painful and create swollen looking fingers and knees, so if you already have either of these ailments, it's important to speak to a physician as you approach menopause.

Bruising may be another symptom as low levels of hormones decreases the skin's ability to retain water, which makes the skin thinner so there is less of a buffer against injury. This leads to more painful and prominent bruising.

Menopausal women may also start to experience more regular hot flashes. Most women get the sensation of heat rising through their body, mainly affecting their chest, neck, and face, causing them to sweat profusely in a short amount of time. If you lose too much body heat from this you may feel a chill once the episode passes. In addition to suddenly feeling very hot, you may experience a rapid heartbeat, and feelings of anxiety, and, if you are of a lighter complexion, you may notice your skin starting to redden. The length of these episodes varies from person to person but on average they last around two to five minutes.

It is not clear exactly how hormonal changes cause hot flashes but most research suggests that they occur when your body's thermostat (hypothalamus) becomes more sensitive to slight changes to body temperature. So, if your hypothalamus senses slight warmth, your body will sweat far too much as an attempt to cool you down. Fortunately, not all women who go through menopause have hot flashes but factors that could increase your risk of having them include smoking, obesity, and sadly race. More Black women have reported hot flashes during menopause than other races, with Asian women experiencing it the least (TED, 2020).

These symptoms can be particularly disheartening as it may make you want to put a halt to some of the activities you enjoy, but this doesn't mean you should live a completely sedentary life. In fact, the opposite is needed to maintain a healthy lifestyle, so it is best to manage the symptoms as best as you can or maybe perform exercise in manageable smaller bursts rather than longer sessions.

No More Periods

If you are further into your menopausal journey, you will not have had a period for some time. You've probably gotten rid of the majority of your sanitary products and are counting down to that 12-month date when you can officially say that you have gone through menopause and come out the other side! Not having a monthly cycle is the most obvious indication that your menopause diagnosis is approaching and it is purely down to our good old friend, estrogen. So little of this hormone is being made in your body that your ovaries stop releasing eggs, so you no longer need to shed the lining of your womb which usually shows up as a period.

If you are closer to the beginning of your menopausal journey, your periods may still be very unpredictable in length, frequency, and flow, so it's best to always have a sanitary pad or panty liner handy, just in case.

Unfortunately, or fortunately (depending on how you view it), there is nothing that can be done to bring your periods back once they've stopped, so I would say to embrace this time and enjoy the absence of cramps, bloating, and breakouts that tend to come with it.

Mental Health Issues

Changes to our mental health can be one of, if not the most difficult symptom of menopause. This is because it is 'invisible' yet all encompassing, so it is very hard for others to understand and support. Menopause can induce stress, anxiety, depression, and fear, as well as memory loss and worry surrounding our mortality. It can feel isolating too, and all of these can have negative effects on how we feel about ourselves.

Depression looks different on everyone but classic signs include feeling tearful, hopeless, or empty. It is more than feeling sad for a few days but rather a persistent low mood that can last for weeks or months. Anxiety is a normal bodily response to a situation in which we feel nervous or apprehensive, but when it is left to its own devices and not managed, it can be crippling. It can make you withdraw from friends and family, make your heart race and palms sweat, and stop you from carrying out your normal daily activities. We can be affected by these mental health issues more during menopause because the same hormones that regulate our menstrual cycle also influence serotonin, which is a chemical found in the brain that promotes feelings of happiness and well-being. The reduction of these hormones, and therefore serotonin, during this time can result in us feeling inconsolably sad and irritable or having regular mood swings.

It is easy to think that our mental wellness starts and ends in the brain but, in female bodies, our brains and our reproductive system actually interact with each other in what is called the neuroendocrine system. This means that the health of one is dependent on the health of the other to a certain extent. For example, when our ovaries start to age and there is a reduction of estrogen, our brain picks up on this and begins to slow down too, so as not to waste this hormone because estrogen is also important in its function and energy. We may therefore start to feel more mentally tired, forgetful, and anxious but rest assured, neuroscientist Lisa Mosconi detected no changes in cognitive behavior during her studies, so we can be just as sharp at problem-solving and performing tasks.

Mosconi also found that memory and mental health may decline faster in women than in men because the hormones we possess have different lifespans. Testosterone, high levels of which are found in men, lasts a very long time so men rarely suffer from any symptoms of decline during their average lifetime. Estrogen, however, will stop working properly after a shorter period of time, so women tend to feel the effect of this on their brains in their 40s or 50s. This suggests that our brains are actually sensitive to hormonal age rather than chronological age, so women who go through menopause younger can still feel the mental symptoms.

This decline in mental energy can make us feel as though we are no longer contributing in our professional or personal lives, especially as, for Black women, there is an idea that we should always be strong, shouldn't show any signs of slowing down, and be the person who fixes everything. It can make us feel as though we don't have the capability to be the leaders we are destined to be, but this is not the case at all. Women over 40 are kicking down barriers and excelling in so many fields, showing that our minds are, and can continue to be, brilliant, both creatively and academically. For example, at age 41, Dr Eve J Hugginbotham was appointed Chair of the Ophthalmology and Visual Science of Maryland School of Medicine. She was the first woman to head a university-based ophthalmology department in the USA and is currently the Vice Dean for diversity and inclusion at the Perelman School of Medicine and a board-certified ophthalmologist. At age 42, filmmaker Ava DuVerney directed the 2015 BET Best Movie, *Selma*, at 49 Viola Davis won an Emmy and novelist Toni Morrison won the Nobel Prize for Literature at age 62. So, you see, being a mature woman doesn't mean that your mind is less capable than the younger generation. In fact, MIT professor Pierre Azoulay's research showed that the average modern business founder is 40 years old and a founder aged 50 is approximately twice as likely to create a successful public business than a 30-year-old (Worthy, 2022). In the past two years of the pandemic, there has also been a boom in entrepreneurship among the average Black women, with 52% of us wanting to leave corporate America to start our own businesses in the next two years (Worthy, 2022). We are the fastest growing group of entrepreneurs, making up 42% of new women-owned businesses, possibly because we have a history of "I'll do it myself" and have often become entrepreneurs out of necessity because of the ongoing wealth gap. So, as long as your keep your mind active and healthy, being menopausal shouldn't stop your desire to achieve.

There are many other menopausal symptoms that your body may experience such as increased urination, insomnia, sensitive breasts, headaches and a racing heart but it is important not to panic because there are both alternative and traditional treatments available for you to use to help you start feeling.

Chapter 3:
Alternative and Natural Treatment

In 2021, it was found that 73% of women reported that they were not treating their current menopause symptoms, despite feeling unhappy (Gordon, 2021). This is such a shame because there are many treatments that can drastically improve your quality of life and if you aren't keen on traditional treatment like hormone replacement therapy, alternative and natural ones are readily accessible.

The Black community has a history of using herbs, spices, and alternative treatments for anything from a cold to an upset stomach. Some African tribes even use a traditional mixture of plant-based medicine and spiritual rituals to treat more serious medical problems such as infertility, heart disease, or depression.

Our relationship with plant medicine predates the first written account in 1500 BCE, in which Ancient Egyptians listed the recipes for over 850 herbal medicines and our knowledge and respect for these natural treatments has traveled with us through history (Ward, 2021). It kept many people alive when traveling across the world during enslavement and later, while escaping plantations with herbalist Harriet Tubman. She used her knowledge of plants and spirituality to keep her passengers of the Underground Railroad safe and then to heal both Black and white soldiers during the Civil War. This interplay between spiritual folk wisdom and Western science continues to inspire us today, with organizations such as Harriet's Apothecary offering customized alternative services to help heal trauma and stress affecting BIPOC individuals.

During 2020, it was found that an increasing amount of Black people started looking for natural healing. Herbalist Jamesa Hawthorne said that more and more of the community were reaching out for her "oatmeal bath for the brain" or "natural immunity builder" as treatment for stress, grief, and fear following the devastating and unprecedented effects of the pandemic as well as the traumatic killings of George Flloyd and Breonna Taylor. She realized that people of color were not only seeking natural remedies because they trusted nature more than they did Western drugs but because they were looking for somewhere to be heard in a place where Black voices usually aren't; the healthcare system. This has led to the uncovering, development, and use of more holistic and alternative treatments for menopause symptoms too and the following are great example but as with any food items or supplements used for medical purposes, it is important to consult your healthcare provider if you have any other underlying conditions that may be affected by their implementation.

For Stronger and Nourished Hair and Nails

Biotin and other B vitamins such as niacin, B12, and folic acid can be used to effectively improve thinning hair and weak nails. You can purchase them as supplements or they can be found naturally in foods such as lentils, liver, nuts, dairy products, and cereal grains. Vitamins A and C, as well as iron and zinc also stimulate hair growth by increasing blood flow to the scalp and improving hair follicle structure. A lack of protein can impact the keratin, so it is advised to eat enough protein-rich fish, red meat, nuts, and leafy greens, such as kale.

Working from the inside out with changes to your diet usually has the best results but there are also things you can start or stop doing to your hair and scalp that will support growth and avoid damage. These include keeping your hair in its natural state as much as possible, as heat from tongs or dryers and chemicals found in relaxers can damage the hair and make it break more and quicker than usual. Staying active can also help as it gets your blood pumping to your scalp and releases oxytocin which relieves stress, both of which regulate your hormones and combat a range of other menopausal symptoms. Staying hydrated, protecting your hair at night and in the sun, and massaging your scalp each week can also be beneficial.

As Black women, we are often guilty of using a lot of products in our hair because afro hair is naturally dry due its curl patterns. This buildup of product can be harmful to the scalp whether you are going through menopause or not, so I recommend doing an apple cider vinegar rinse once or twice a month to cleanse the pores in the scalp or a witch-hazel wipe of the hairline 5–10 minutes before shampooing to reduce inflammation or irritation. Remember to condition afterwards as both products have a drying effect.

If you feel as though you are already really struggling with mental and physical effects of hair loss, of course, please don't suffer in silence or feel as though you must push through if it is damaging your confidence and self-esteem. There is no shame in doing what you need to do to feel and look the way you want to, so you may want to consider some tricks to make your hair look fuller. You could add color, which makes your strands look thicker, try a short haircut with layering, or even go the extra mile and purchase a fabulous wig and try out styles you'd never been able to before!

For Glowing and Supple Skin

By eating foods that are rich in vitamin C and sulfur, you will help your body make more collagen. This includes red peppers, strawberries, guava, and kale for vitamin C and broccoli, cauliflower, and garlic for sulfur. Bone broth is also a direct source of collagen, which is thankfully something used in a lot of Caribbean and African American cooking already. Alongside a balanced diet of oily fish such as salmon, you may also consider taking a good omega-3 supplement. It includes eicosapentaenoic acid (EPA) which regulates oil production, blocks enzymes that reduce collagen levels, works as an antioxidant, and helps repair and protect damaged skin.

Drinking water is the best way to keep your skin hydrated from the inside, so be sure to drink enough throughout the day and apply moisturizer immediately after a bath or shower. When bathing, it's best to use soaps, gels, lotions, and other skin care products that contain low amounts or no chemical ingredients that remove the natural oils from your skin; you should try to use ones that contain shea butter or coconut oil instead. You could even add a scoop of oatmeal to your bath as it contains soothing plant chemicals called avenanthramides that help reduce itching and inflammation. The lactic acid in milk is another skin soother, so you could try patting your skin with a cloth soaked in milk for some relief from dryness or itching. Although water is great on the inside, on the outside of our bodies, it can have a drying effect, so reducing shower or bath times and using lukewarm water instead of hot can help minimize this.

For moisturization, natural products that contain macadamia, apricot, or coconut oil are great because they are rich sources of omega 7, vitamins E and B, fatty acids, and proteins that can penetrate the skin and nourish the lower layers. Beeswax is a natural way to protect the skin from environmental damage by forming a protective barrier, so remember to apply this last.

Even though many Black people have highly melanated skin compared to that of non-Black people, it is still important to wear sunscreen, even when the sun seems to be hidden by clouds. Understandably, there is a reluctance to use sun protective cream in the Black community because the majority of products are not formulated to be optimal or attractive on those with darker skin tones. They often leave us looking gray and/or shiny, so, despite its importance, some of us will avoid using them. Fortunately, there are a few black-owned brands who have tackled this issue with a range of products that don't create this ghostly cast, so why not try products such as Broad Spectrum's Black Girl Sunscreen, No Shade Sunscreen Oil by Mele or Fenty Skin's Hydra Vizor sunscreen moisturizer, as recommended by Michelle Henry, a board-certified dermatologist and clinical instructor of dermatology at Weill Medical College?

All of these tips can help you return to or maintain that "Black don't crack" complexion and reduce the appearance of "menopausal skin".

For Weight-Loss and Body Sculpting

Naturally, weight loss starts with your diet. At whatever age you are, eating healthily and moving more will generally help you to reduce the fat stored in your body, so it is valuable to eat fresh fruit and vegetables rather than fast food and takeaways. Due to their low-calorie count, you can eat large amounts of grapes, apples, carrots, and broccoli to feel full and it will still be beneficial for your weight loss journey, while keeping you nourished and healthy. There are also some household herbs and spices that can help you to lose overall weight but don't attempt to eat them on their own for a miraculous speedy weight loss because after all, slow and steady wins the race!

Fenugreek, a spice derived from a plant belonging to the legume family, is found to help control appetite, therefore reducing food intake and supporting weight loss. Just supplementing 8 grams of fenugreek fiber daily was shown to increase feelings of fullness. Cayenne pepper is a spice that contains capsaicin which can slightly boost metabolism, reduce hunger, and increase feelings of fullness too, due to its ability to reduce the levels of ghrelin; the hormone responsible for stimulating hunger. The oregano herb contains carvacrol which is a powerful compound that controls fat synthesis in the body. Human-based research is lacking however, but it has been tested on mice and had a positive effect for body weight loss, even when on a high-fat diet.

Cinnamon is an aromatic spice that is rich in antioxidants and some studies have found that it could increase weight loss. It has been found to be especially effective in stabilizing blood sugar, which can help reduce appetite and hunger. It also decreases levels of digestive enzymes to slow the breakdown of carbohydrates, making you feel fuller for longer. There are also benefits with cumin, black pepper, turmeric, cardamon, and more, so a well spiced healthy meal seems to be the way forward. Just avoid adding too many fats, oils, and salt to your food as this can have the opposite effect.

Exercise is also important for body sculpting and removing that 'menopot' layer of fat around the abdomen. It is key to remember however, that you cannot target fat loss i.e., you can't simply practice abdominal exercises and lose fat in this area alone. Your body will lose fat proportionately across your entire body and unfortunately the stomach is usually the last place that it disappears as this area contains 'stubborn' fat. So, creating a varied and consistent workout plan is best and you are bound to notice an overall difference within a few months if your diet is also monitored.

It will also be beneficial to include some resistance training in your regimen to build muscle so that your metabolism increases. This means that you will be burning more calories even when in a rested state. You can also use weight training to sculpt your body. For example, if you'd like thicker thighs and a smaller waist, you could perform squats and abdominal crunches to grow or tighten these areas. When you introduce this type of training into your routine, you may notice an increase in weight initially, but this will just be your muscle growing rather than fat accumulating, so try to focus less on what you weigh and more on how you look and feel.

For Increased Sex Drive

Topical vitamin E oil applied to the vagina can reduce vaginal dryness (and even hot flashes), making sex feel more comfortable. Normally, the vagina stays lubricated with natural clear fluids but the drop in estrogen levels can reduce this significantly so you may want to try alternatives like this to make sex more enjoyable. This can help return your sex drive to what's normal for you.

Herbs and spices such as cloves, maca, ginger, fennel, saffron, and nutmeg, can not only heat up your food but also your sex life as they contain nutrients that stimulate blood flow and lubrication in all the right places. Fennel in particular was used by ancient Egyptians to boost a woman's libido and for good reason, as it has estrogenic effects and can even help relieve menstrual cramps, so having these as supplements or using the real deal in food can often help.

There are, however, some natural aphrodisiac supplements that have been passed down through the ages and have the opposite effect or induce negative side-effects so you should steer clear of them. For example, yohimbine (or yohimbe) supplements, despite their popularity, are said to be potentially harmful and have been banned in several countries. Spanish fly should also be avoided due to its potentially dangerous side effects such as difficulty swallowing, nausea, vomiting blood, and painful urination. Its use dates back to Roman times where empresses and gladiators would use it to have orgies or spice up their affairs. The original supplement was created from crushed blister beetles and contains cantharidin, which actually led to unhealthy inflammation and swelling of the genitals, not attraction or arousal as they had once thought! Today, although many products advertised as Spanish fly, they are often not the real extracts and rather a mixture of different herbs, water, and spices, so always check the labels. "Mad honey" and bufo toad were also considered natural aphrodisiacs but both can adversely affect your long-term health.

It is well known that oysters have aphrodisiac properties and this is because of their high zinc content and these are perfectly safe when cooked properly. This compound increases blood flow which can help it get to those vital sex organs. Oysters contain more zinc than any other food source with just one serving providing 673% of your daily value (Roth, 2016), but if you aren't a fan of their texture, like many of us, you can try lobster or crab instead.

Surprisingly, the humble apple can also play a role in improving your sex drive as they are rich in a compound called quercetin, which is an antioxidant that promotes circulation and lowers blood pressure. High blood pressure can lead to sexual disinterest because it can cause fatigue and your body will find it harder to respond to sexual activity.

If you are open to it, acupuncture or massage may be a potential method for boosting sex drive in women. They can help reduce anxiety, stress, and insomnia which can all be underlying causes of a decreased libido.

Finally, there's no better aphrodisiac than confidence! By improving the way you feel about your body, and yourself in general, you are bound to feel more sexy inside and out. So why not try a few positive affirmations that tell you exactly how sexual and sensual you are and even get a partner involved over course of the day to really get those juices flowing!

For Physical Discomfort

Soy (food form not tablets), flaxseed, red clover, and evening primrose oil are good for treating hot flashes and night sweats. In fact, in a recent study a combination of dong quai and these other herbs was proven to significantly reduce them (Hill, 2020). The herb black cohosh has also recently received a lot of attention for its possible prevention of hot flashes but because it has some links to liver problems, it is best to check with your healthcare provider before you start to use it medicinally. It is also best to avoid caffeine and alcohol as these can increase your body temperature, so stick to cold water or juices for some consistent relief.

For aches and pains, maintaining a healthy weight will stop extra stress being placed on your joints and tendons and following an anti-inflammatory diet full of oily fish, nuts, and seeds will also help. As well as this, vitamin D supplements can be helpful as it regulates the amount of calcium and phosphate in the body, keeping bones, joints, teeth, and muscles healthy and pain free. It is created naturally in the body when sunlight is absorbed through our skin but if you have a darker complexion, the sun's rays take longer to penetrate and create this useful vitamin. So, if you are a Black person living in a country that has a low amount of sunlight, or you spend a lot of time inside, you may not be getting the amount your body needs to function well. This means that taking supplements is very important, as it is only found in a small number of foods such as oily fish (salmon, sardines, herring, and mackerel), red meat, liver, and egg yolks, and it is difficult to get a sufficient dosage of vitamin D from these alone.

Massage is another great way to combat the physical discomfort you may feel during menopause. Manipulating the muscle tissue and skin in a relaxing or stimulating way can ease knots, induce sleep, and help produce chemicals in the body that make you feel good, not only physically but also mentally.

For A Healthy Mind, Body, and Soul

Now that we've taken care of our outer bodies, it's important and necessary to look after our inner selves too. Our mind and souls will go through a lot during this time of life, so we need to do what we can to ease the mental burden as well.

Exercise

Whether it's dancing, walking, running, kayaking, or roller skating, moving more is proven to improve your mood because exercise releases endorphins into your body, which is a chemical produced by the brain that makes you feel happier, more relaxed, and less anxious. It decreases stress by stimulating the production of neurohormones which improves cognition and mood and if you take part in activities that require coordination, it can boost your brain functionality and memory as it stimulates the growth of new brain cells and prevents age-related decline.

It may seem strange that using energy in this way can give you more energy in return too, but it's true. Getting your heart racing and lungs working will make you feel more energetic in the long term because you will become fitter and want to move around more. Exercise and physical activity can also be social and being around like-minded people can make you feel motivated and positive.

A recent study by Harvard TH Chan School of Public Health found that running for just 15 minutes or walking for one hour per day reduces the risk of major depression by a huge 26%, which is just as effective as antidepressant medication but without the side-effects. You can also use it to treat anxiety through exercise mindfulness which is a practice that involves staying present in the moment.

Paying attention to the sensation of your feet hitting the ground or the rhythm of your breathing—really focusing on the way your body feels when moving—will interrupt the constant worries running through your mind.

In general, the US Department of Health and Human Services recommends that healthy adults try to get at least 150 minutes of moderate aerobic activity, such as brisk walking, cycling, or swimming or 75 minutes of intense activity such as running, heavy yard work, or dancing each week, to maintain health and fitness. You will surely feel the benefits in your mind, body, and soul and you may even discover a hidden talent!

Yoga

Practicing yoga not only helps you with flexibility, strength, and balance but it can help you to improve your mood. It is a group of physical, mental, and spiritual practices that originated in ancient India which aim to control and still the mind.

Black women have historically used it as a tool for healing from our disproportionate exposure to anxiety, stress, depression, and heart disease. It is often practiced in safe spaces and with niche types such as trap or hip-hop yoga growing it is becoming increasingly popular in our community. This means that yoga can also be used to connect with fellow sisters who can help distract you from the symptoms of menopause or even provide you with a listening ear. While the majority of yoga practitioners are white in the US, the percentage of Black yogis has slightly increased from 3% to more than 5% since 2012 (Jean, 2020), so there is a growing community out there for you to take comfort in.

Activist Angela Davis has spoken about participating in yoga, saying that it gave her a sense of peace after her 1970 arrest (Jean, 2020).

She states that it prepared her for struggle while in prison, made her more energetic, and helped her learn about the need for self-care. Rosa Parks' niece also recounts her aunt valuing yoga as a way of clearing her mind and keeping her body limber with the goal of living a longer and fuller life and the Rosa and Raymond Parks Institute of Self-Development, which implements yoga and meditation, was even created and to encourage other Black women to do the same.

Breathing Exercises and Meditation

It may seem simple but, inhaling and exhaling in a smooth and controlled way can really improve your mental state. It can be performed during a full meditation session or used when out and about to bring you back to a state of calm.

Meditation is a simple, fast, and inexpensive way to reduce stress. It has been practiced for thousands of years, originally used to help deepen the understanding of sacred forces but today, it is commonly used for relaxation. Organizations such as Black Girl in Om, Liberate Meditation, or Black Zen which have been created to cater to women of color in particular all recognize its power and benefits for our community and provide safe spaces to meditate in but of course, it can be done on your own in your home, car, or studio.

You can try taking part in guided meditation, sometimes called guided visualization, which encourages you to form mental images of places or situations you find relaxing, such as being on a beach vacation. While doing this, you or your teacher can introduce smells, sights, sounds, and textures, so that as many of your senses are involved as possible, making it feel real. For example, playing the sound of waves lapping the shore, smelling salted water, and running your fingers through a bowl of sand can really place you in the scenario in your mind and help you to still reap the benefits of this vacation wherever you are.

Mantra or transcendental meditation is when you silently repeat a calming word, thought, or phase to prevent distracting thoughts and boost your mood. For example, saying "I am at peace with my life" or "My body is in control" to yourself repetitively will eventually make you believe it and feel less worried or anxious.

Mindfulness meditation is about having increased awareness and acceptance of the present. You are encouraged to sit quietly and only focus on what is happening in that exact moment; the sounds you hear, the fragrances you smell, and the sensations in your body. This will be difficult at first but the more you do it, the more your physical and emotional health will improve. It is often practiced during yoga but can be used in isolation or as part of cognitive behavioral therapy. It is a great way to check in with your body for any new menopausal symptoms that you need to address and give yourself the much-needed attention you may not be getting from the outside world.

Cognitive Behavioral Therapy

Cognitive Behavioral Therapy (CBT) is a psychological treatment that helps you to manage any of your life problems. You would work with a therapist to change the way you think and behave in certain situations so that you can feel more positive and are able to find solutions quicker. For example, when going through menopause and experiencing forgetfulness, instead of beating yourself up about it and questioning your capabilities, you would be encouraged to take a moment to pause, accept what you have forgotten and move on, while reassuring yourself that you will find a new solution without the item or knowledge you've forgotten. This way of thinking helps to break the negative cycles that induce anxiety and depression and will eventually lead to a more positive outlook on life.

Sadly however, it has been passed around within the Black community that we don't or shouldn't go to therapy. This is usually because of the many barriers that make it less accessible or appealing to us. For example, professional therapy can often be expensive and despite the Affordable Care Act, mental health care is not usually covered by insurance or has high co-pays and unaffordable deductibles. It is therefore preferred to spend money on more immediate needs like food or bills, leaving our mental health neglected. There is also familial shame and cultural stigma around mental illness among Black people, with a 2014 study showing that 63% of Black people believe that having a mental health issue is a sign of weakness (Femestella, 2022), therefore, going to therapy is seen as acceptance of a problem you 'shouldn't' have. The lack of diversity in the mental health care system, distrust in the medical industry, and negative past experiences are also factors but, thankfully this perception is changing.

Celebrities such as Taraji P Henson, Gabrielle Union, Hallie Berry, and Kerry Washington have all openly discussed their participation in therapy and endorse it for achieving positive and helpful solutions to their struggles. Washington says that her brain and heart are important to her, so doesn't think twice about looking after them as she would do her teeth. Henson values professional therapists because they can give you helpful exercises that friends can't, so that when you are on a 'ledge' you have "things to say to yourself that will get you off that ledge and past your weakest moments" (Femestella, 2022). This is exactly how CBT works so I urge you to join these powerful Black women in their quest for mental stability during such a turbulent time of your life.

Hypnotherapy

Words can be powerful and if you are open to it, the words of a hypnotherapist can truly change your life. Hypnotherapy is when you are put into a very relaxed and almost trance-like state and are given repetitive and influential verbal cues by the therapist. They would encourage you to be open to change or improvement and it is said that doing this while in a hypnotic state is more effective than while in your normal state. It requires a lot of trust and there is some skepticism around this practice but when fully understood and embraced it can truly work.

As much as the media has led you to believe it, true hypnosis doesn't involve swaying pocket watches and embarrassing acts. You are completely in control of your body during hypnosis, as it is closer to a feeling of intense concentration and focus which will make your senses and mind more open. It can help plant seeds of inspiration in your mind, declutter your thoughts, and bring about feelings of acceptance and satisfaction.

It is important to note that hypnotherapy doesn't work on everyone, with studies showing that only 10% of the population is highly hypnotizable (Holland, 2018) but if you struggle with talking therapies such as CBT this might be a good option to try instead.

Massage Therapy and Aromatherapy

The muscle manipulation, stimulation, and relaxation induced through massage therapy and aromatherapy is highly beneficial during menopause. This is because it gives your body a boost of endorphins that can be incredibly grounding and prevent or ease anxiety building up. From a spiritual perspective, massage can also be used to take care of our souls. It has been used by ancient civilizations right up to the present day to reset, cleanse, and balance our energy, making us feel happier and more at peace holistically.

Aromatherapy, which is the use of essential oils extracted from plants, can naturally help improve anxiety and insomnia too. It is considered as an alternative treatment but now that the oils are more accessible and affordable, it is growing in popularity and becoming more mainstream. You can apply small quantities of the oils to your body, add a few drops to a warm bath, or use scented candles or incense around the house to fill your rooms with a beautiful fragrance, like lavender, to help you to relax. The smells stimulate your limbic system which is connected to your memories and emotions, so if you use a particular fragrance during a positive time, when you smell it again it will remind you of this time and make you feel good all over again.

Food and Drink

Drinks such as chamomile tea can help to calm the mind and fresh fruit, vegetables, and 'good' fats are also important for positive mental health. Having a well-balanced diet can make us feel more alert, and counterbalance the slowing effects menopause has on the brain. An inadequate, processed food diet on the other hand can leave you feeling fatigued, impair decision making, and slow down your reaction time. The sugar found in these unhealthy foods often leads to inflammation throughout the body and the brain which can also induce mood disorders. Instead, you should try to eat more complex carbohydrates such as brown rice, quinoa, beets and sweet potatoes, as well as lean proteins and fatty acids found in eggs, chicken, fish, and soybeans.

The old adage that you are what you eat is, in this case, true, with researchers proving that there is a connection between your gut and your brain. They are physically linked by the vagus nerve so your gut has the ability to influence the emotional behavior of your brain and the brain can alter the type of bacteria living in the gut. This means that being mindful of what you put into your body is very important when trying to regulate your mental health. There is no doubt that processed fast food is highly addictive, but if you can go through your menopausal years without it, you will certainly feel the difference in many aspects of your life.

All of these treatments can be used instead of traditional medicines or as well as, but if there is any symptoms you are particularly concerned about during your menopause, I urge you to speak to your health care professional.

Chapter 4:
Professional Support and Traditional Treatment

Mainstream medicine certainly has its place when treating menopause symptoms. It can be used alone or alongside other complimentary treatments such as massage, CBT, herbs, and hypnotherapy but doctors tend to prefer more traditional treatment for menopause and it may indeed be the best option in some cases.

When To Seek Professional Support

Experiencing symptoms when going through menopause is very common, so it is considered normal; over 85% of women have symptoms (Forbes, 2021). But if your symptoms are particularly bad and don't seem to be improving with alternative treatment, then you may need to get some professional support through Western medicine. This can feel a little overwhelming if you are used to taking care of yourself but in order to have a smooth transition into menopause and a comfortable journey through it, it will probably be for the best in the case of extreme or unexpected symptoms.

Extreme symptoms include any of the common symptoms of menopause occurring in a way that interferes with your daily life. For example, if you are unable to go to work or feel unwell regularly. Unexpected symptoms included a lot of weight gain, dizziness, or increased anxiety so in these cases it is usually worth involving your doctor to at least weigh up your options.

It is also necessary to get professional support if you start experiencing symptoms before the age of 45 or if you experience vaginal bleeding after menopause. Menopause is a time when you could also be at a higher risk of hypertension, cholesterol disorder, osteoporosis and diabetes, so even if you plan to use alternative therapy, seeking professional advice should be considered.

Trusting Your Doctor

If the 2020 Covid-19 pandemic has shown us anything, it is that there is a mistrust in traditional medical care among Black people. Despite knowing that African Americans were more likely to get seriously ill or die from the virus, we were the least likely to take the vaccine.

This mistrust is completely understandable because we have a long history of poor, humiliating, or non-existent treatment in so many aspects of healthcare including childbirth, vaccination, HIV treatment, cancer, and substance use disorder. Enslaved Africans even faced gruesome experiments such as forced sterilization at the hands of white medical professionals, so it is little wonder why 42% of Black American said they would be unwilling to take the Covid-19 vaccine in November 2020 and 55% say they distrust the healthcare system in general (Hostetter & Klein, 2021). We have been undertreated for pain due to false beliefs about our biological differences and a poll taken in October 2020 showed that 7 out of 10 Black Americans felt that they had been treated unfairly in a medical setting. When it comes to menopause specifically, it also doesn't help that 32% of women say they feel as though their doctor isn't comfortable talking about menopause, causing them to look for support elsewhere (Forbes, 2021)!

Thankfully, with these shocking statistics and the resurgence of the Black Lives Matter movement in mind, health systems are working harder to reduce health disparities by confronting institutional racism head on. Many health authorities have committed to treating patients as experts on their own bodies and trusting them when they feel a serious or persistent problem. For example, the Merck for Mothers initiative was set up with the aim of reducing maternal mortality worldwide by doing this. Many organizations have also committed to using more empathy by partnering with research sites in minority communities which will help them to understand the challenges and history of medical care for Black and Latino people. They will use these outreach exercises to hear and validate the concerns we have but also dispel any hindering myths that are stopping us from attaining the treatment we need. Building relationships outside of the exam rooms like this is also an initiative programs like 3rd Conversation are implementing, by creating a space for patients to talk to healthcare providers and find solutions together, so that minorities feel more in control of their treatment.

These feelings of mistrust cannot be removed overnight and there is still a need for more changes to overcome institutional racism but it is reassuring to see that steps are being taken so that women like me can feel comfortable in receiving the treatment we deserve and so often require. Michelle Morse MD MPH, former co-chair of Brigham and Women's Hospital Health Equity Committee, said "After much conversation and debate, the concept of institutional racism was no longer distant, abstract, or someone else's problem" so there is a definite ongoing shift in the status quo when it comes to what is required in healthcare for Black people.

Preparing For an Appointment

If you decide to go ahead with seeing a professional about the option of starting traditional treatment, being prepared for your appointment can really help calm your anxiety or ease any feelings of uncertainty around it, so here are a few tips that can make you feel more at ease.

If your provider offers double appointments, it could be a good idea to book one so that you have enough time to discuss your symptoms in detail and address all the concerns you have. Before the appointment, take a look through the list of possible menopausal symptoms and record any that you are experiencing and when. It will also be useful to make a note of any changes to your monthly cycle, any questions you have and any medication you are taking, including herbal supplements. If you are particularly anxious you can always bring a friend or family member along with you for support if your practice allows this.

During your appointment your doctor should discuss the stages of menopause, common symptoms, how menopause is diagnosed, lifestyle changes, benefits and risks of treatment, and how menopause can affect your future health. They may also carry out blood tests to check your hormone levels or to rule out any underlying issues but most women can start treatment without this. While you're there, try to be bold and mature when talking about your body, especially when it comes to your more intimate areas. Dr Rosalind Jackson (also known as Dr Roz), a Black OB/GYN who has been practicing for over 18 years, recalls having so many women attend appointments with her not being able to even say the word 'vagina.' In her 2017 TED Talk, *The Woman You Become*, she tells us that some of her female patients visit her and say "Alice doesn't feel well" or refer to their vaginas as "vajay-jays" or "lady parts" and she finds it hilarious but also worrying! How can it be a part of the body that all females have but we are ashamed or embarrassed to simply say the name of it? We should be comfortable with every inch of our bodies and that includes the vagina, labia, and clitoris.

When it comes to the end of the appointment, try not to leave the room with any of your questions unanswered. This will avoid any confusion or further anxiety and don't be afraid to get a second opinion if you aren't confident in what you were told.

In most cases, your doctor will prescribe hormone replacement therapy (HRT) but if they don't and it's something you want, it is important to know your rights as a patient. If you can show that you are fully informed, understand any risks, and can clearly explain that you still wish to have HRT treatment, your doctor is more likely to consider your views seriously.

Hormone Replacement Therapy

The most popular form of traditional treatment for menopause symptoms is hormone replacement therapy (HRT). Essentially, it replaces the hormones that have been reduced. It is very effective at relieving hot flashes, night sweats, mood swings, vaginal dryness, and reduced sex drive, so many women choose to use and benefit from it as a one-stop fix. It can also be used to treat osteoporosis (weak bones) which can develop during menopause.

If you decide to go down this route, speak to your doctor as soon as you start experiencing symptoms and they will start you on a low dosage, increasing it if and when they need to. It will usually take a few weeks to feel the difference and doctors recommend trying it for approximately three months to determine whether it is the right treatment for you. It is safe for most women but if you have a history of breast, ovarian or womb cancer, blood clots, high blood pressure, or liver disease you may be advised to try a different type of treatment or will be monitored more closely.

Like any other medical treatment, HRT does come with some possible side-effects which includes tender breasts, headaches, nausea, indigestion, and vaginal bleeding but the benefits outweigh the risks, especially if you are suffering from many severe symptoms of menopause. It's also worth noting that you can still get pregnant while using hormone replacement therapy so, if you are sexually active and don't want children, remember to use contraception for at least two years after your last period if you are under 50 or a year if you are over 50, to avoid any unplanned surprises!

Types of HRT

There are two types of hormone replacement therapy that are usually given to menopausal women. Combined; a mixture of estrogen and progestogen, and estrogen only, which is mainly used for women who have had a hysterectomy, like myself. Taking the combined treatment if you have a womb is important because the estrogen makes the lining of the womb build up which can increase your risk of cancer but the progestogen prevents too much build up, thus reducing the risk.

The optimal estrogen in HRT is a type called 17 beta oestradiol which is identical to the estrogen found in the body, in that it has the same molecular structure, so it is often considered natural but it is derived from a plant chemical that is extracted from yam plants. The optimal type of progestogen is called micronized progesterone and this is also the body identical version and using this type is usually associated with fewer side effects than other types. The hormone testosterone can also be prescribed to improve mood, energy, stamina, motivation, and libido.

HRT treatment comes in a variety of forms which you can choose based on your preference and its effectiveness for you. You can take tablets, use patches, apply gels or creams to your vagina, or insert pessaries or rings. Your plan can also be either constant or in cycles, much like the contraceptive pill, so all of these options mean that your HRT can be altered to suit your individual health needs.

Other Prescribed Treatments

Despite its benefits, there has been quite a lot of resistance to using HRT because of the research published in 2002, which found that HRT presented more health risks than benefits. After a reanalysis it was revealed that there were limitations in this research and it was in fact safe to use when prescribed correctly. This revelation seems to still not have settled many women's nerves around its use, with 65% of women in a Bonafide survey saying that they would not consider using it unless their healthcare provider specifically recommended it or a new clinical study emerged proving its safety again.

Although it is technically another type of hormone therapy, the use of tibolone could be considered as an alternative to estrogen. However, it hasn't been researched as extensively as some other forms of therapy, so additional advice is recommended. Antidepressants are another non-estrogen treatment used for hot flashes. The selective serotonin receptor inhibitors (SSRIs) are the most common type and it is the only non-hormonal therapy specifically approved for hot flashes in the United States.

Whatever type of treatment you decide to go for, if any, know that you deserve to live a fulfilling, open, and happy life.

Chapter 5:
Living Your Best Life with Menopause

According to a Female Founders Fund survey from 2020, 78% of women said that menopause had interfered with their lives (Gordon, 2021), but with treatment, practical tips, support from friends, family, and colleagues when you need it, and a sense of humor, day-to-day life can return to 'normal'. In fact, you should try to live your best life during menopause and these tips can help you on your way.

An Inspiring Morning Routine

When you wake up, you may realize that you've had a bit of a sweaty night. The sheets may be a little damp and your partner may have been kicked a few times while you were tossing and turning but there are a few ways to help kickstart your day in the right direction.

1. **Keep a towel handy**. You may have experienced night sweats, so having a small towel by your bed can help you to mop up a sweaty face, neck, or chest when you wake up.

2. **Practice positive affirmations**. Speaking positivity into your day and mind will help you feel motivated and energized. Find a few statements that resonate with you and repeat them out loud several times while looking into a mirror. Imagine the statements to be completely true and say them with confidence and they will be something to remember if you experience any anxiety or low mood during the day. You could even write the affirmations down and keep them with you in a small notebook or diary.

3. **Have a quick wash and moisturize well**. Being quick in the shower or bath will stop your skin from drying out. Applying creams or lotions to your body straight after will then help to seal in the moisture and leave your skin feeling soft and supple. Natural oils or butters such as coconut or shea are ideal but a heavier cream can also be great for menopausal skin. You may want to use a lighter lotion on your face to avoid build up and the potential of breakouts.

4. **Slow down**. Waking up with enough time to get ready will stop you from rushing and lessen the chances of you getting hot and bothered. So set your alarm approximately 30 minutes earlier than

usual, so that you can then take your time, keep cool, and enjoy getting ready slowly.

5. **Wear layers**. Instead of wearing a thick jumper in the winter months, it is wiser to wear layers. For example, you could wear a tank top and a shirt with a sweatshirt on top, so that if you do experience hot flashes, you won't have to strip down to your underwear to feel some relief. Carrying a spare loose shirt in summer months may also be reassuring for you if you are worried about sweat patches but if you must wear a heavier long-sleeved shirt, a clever trick is to stick a panty liner to the inside where you are prone to patches. The liner will soak up the sweat and nobody will know!

6. **Prepare your meals and supplements for the week**. Preparing and planning your diet will ensure that you are eating more healthily and not snacking on fast food. It will also save you money, so when you cook, try to make enough for the working week, freezing portions where necessary. Keeping your supplements with your food will also make sure you remember to take them each day.

7. **Write a to-do list**. With our hormones making our minds a bit fuzzy, writing a list of what you want

to achieve can be a great way to map out your day and avoid forgetting anything important. It will also help you to prioritize and manage your expectations so you don't feel too overwhelmed. There's also nothing more satisfying than a completed list!

Support At Work

Unless you are fortunate enough to not need to work, you are likely to have a career that requires you to show up and perform at your best every day. Unfortunately, menopause often intersects with critical stages in our careers when many women are moving into leadership positions. Experiencing menopausal symptoms during this time can make it difficult to perform well but there are always solutions to help you get through those all-important hours.

1. **Open up**. If you feel comfortable, tell your colleagues or managers that you are going through menopausal symptoms. Understandably, some women feel uncomfortable doing this because of the current stigma surrounding it, but the more we talk about it, the less taboo it will feel. You may also be helping future generations of menopausal women by getting policies put in place or raising awareness of how it affects our work lives. So, get

the dialogue going about it and educate your employers about what it means for you.

2. **Offer solutions**. If your workplace isn't forthcoming with ways to improve your working environment for yourself and any other women going through menopause, you could also offer practical solutions or adjustments to make it more comfortable. You could suggest moving your desk to a location closer to a window or requesting a fan if you are suffering from hot flashes. Simple things like this can make a big difference and make you more productive, which I'm sure your managers will appreciate.

3. **Take the breaks you are entitled to**. If you suffer from brain fog, splitting your day up into chunks can give your brain a chance to adjust and reset. Working long hours non-stop can fatigue your mind and body so breaks will help you to avoid overwhelm.

4. **Use digital planning tools**. Forgetfulness is an annoying symptom of menopause, so why not use apps such as Trello or Monday to plan your daily, weekly, or even monthly tasks. You can list your du-

ties based on priority, share them with your colleagues, and shift tasks around based on your schedule, all on a platform that is a little more reliable than your brain at the moment.

A Colorful Social Life

Keeping busy and being around people you like can provide a welcome distraction from the symptoms you are struggling with. Being social can also help you understand that you are not alone in what you are experiencing, providing a sense of comfort.

1. **Plan something fun**. On some evenings, organize a meal or outing with someone you enjoy being around. It will give you something to look forward to and focus on as a 'reward' for all of your hard work in the days before.

2. **It's good to talk.** Meet up with people you trust who may be going through the same things as you and simply catch up. Compare experiences or discuss solutions and treatments that work with you, because after all, sharing is caring!

3. **Join support groups**. If you don't have any friends or family members who can empathize with

your menopausal journey, attending support sessions or joining community groups can be a great way to get the feedback and comradery you desire. Groups like Peanut Menopause, Menopause Matters, or Red Hot Mamas can be life-savers and also provide a lot of resources for you to learn from.

4. **Attend group sessions at the gym**. Having a realistic work-out regimen is essential for seeing and feeling the benefits of exercise. By signing up to group sessions, not only will you enjoy the company, but you will also be held accountable by your instructor or fellow gym-goers, meaning that you are more likely to attend and reap the benefits.

5. **Reduce your social media time**. Although our demographic isn't necessarily spending the most amount of time on apps such as Instagram, Twitter, or Tik Tok, being on these addictive platforms can make comparison rear its ugly head. While scrolling through, we may end up seeing hundreds of menopausal or pre-menopausal women who have sweat free brows, are in great shape and are full of energy which can make us feel less than, as we start to wonder why we aren't the feeling and looking same. This can be damaging to your self-esteem, so it will be helpful to limit the time spent using these

apps and it's important to remember that what you see online isn't always the full truth. Rest assured that how you look and feel is usually completely normal and common, you're just seeing other women's highlight reels and not the real life that happens behind the camera.

6. **Start dating**. If you are single and are looking for a relationship or companionship, now is the time to put yourself out there. You know what you want and need and deserve to have a special someone to spend time with. Going through menopause shouldn't stop you from finding romance and happiness and a good partner will be respectful and empathetic. So go for it–it's never too late to find love and seeing who's out there may excite you enough to get your libido back!

7. **Treat yourself**. Let's face it, we work hard and Black women have been through a lot to get to where we are today, collectively and individually. So giving yourself some TLC or treating yourself to something you've wanted for a while will boost your mood, by getting those endorphins flowing and making yourself feel inspired to continue the hard work.

8. **Spend time in nature**. Statistics suggest that Black Americans don't go out into nature as much as other ethnicities but being around trees, plants, water, and animals has been proven to improve your mental health. So instead of having a city break, why not schedule some time in a park or leafy area, switch off your phone (if safe to do so), and enjoy what Mother Nature has to offer. It doesn't mean you have to hug trees or run barefoot into a forest but just looking at and listening to the world around you will benefit your mind, body, and soul tremendously. Being outside also exposes you to more sunlight, which, as we know, will help the valuable production of vitamin D. Organizations such as Outdoor Afro have even been set up to dispel the myth that Black people don't or shouldn't have a relationship with the outdoors and lead fishing excursions, camping trips, and hikes in safe and welcoming environments, so why not give it a try.

9. **Try something you've never done before**. This can give you a sense of achievement and make you feel youthful and energized. Take that trip to Europe, learn a new language, or start your own business. Now is the time!

A Calming Nighttime Routine

Getting a good night's rest can make all the difference when it comes to making the most of the next day. You'll awaken feeling more rested, refreshed, and ready to enjoy what the day has to offer.

1. **Practice yoga, meditation, or stretches.** Gentle movement before bed can help slow down a racing mind and ease any sore muscles. Yoga is a great way to release everything you've been holding onto mentally and physically, meditation can enhance your inner peace and stretching can improve the quality of your sleep. A good stretch for this time is the bear hug, where you stand with your feet hip-width apart and arms open wide. Then cross one arm over the other at the elbows and reach over and grasp the backs of the shoulders. Gently pull your shoulders forward and hold for 20 seconds while breathing deeply. You may want to also try head rolls to relieve tension in your neck, shoulders and upper back, which is where we hold onto a lot of our stress.

2. **Switch off electronic devices an hour before.** In 2011, the National Sleep Foundation found that roughly four in 10 Americans bring their cell phones into bed with them and six out of 10 claimed

to use a computer within one hour of going to bed (Pacheco, 2022). The back-light on these electronic devices can interfere with sleep by suppressing the production of melatonin, a hormone that induces tiredness, so it's not the best practice if you suffer from menopausal insomnia.

3. **Have a glass of water by the bed**. Dehydration can make sleep near impossible. Drinking water before you go to bed can also help you to attain the drop in core body temperature that is required to induce sleep. Having an icy glass nearby can make it easier for you to quench your thirst during the night and cool you down if you have night sweats.

4. **Put a towel down and use some talc**. If night sweats are a regular occurrence for you, laying an old towel under you in bed can help to soak up the sweat and save your sheets. You could also try using some talc powder on your neck and chest, using bedsheets and nightwear made from a lighter material, or keeping a window slightly open overnight.

5. **Purchase some cooling gadgets**. Neck tubes are like the neck supports you wear on long journeys to stop your head from rolling if you fall asleep, but colder. Simply put them in the freezer

for 20 minutes before you go to bed and then place them around your neck. The gel inside will stay cold and cool you down for up to two hours helping you drift off to sleep and avoid night sweats. If you really want to turn up the tech, thermal wristbands are a very fancy way to beat these unpleasant sweats. They are worn on your wrist like a watch and whenever you feel overly warm, you press a button to release a thermal sensation. Fascinatingly, this will help cool the rest of your body by targeting the temperature-sensitive skin on the wrist that helps regulate your body temperature.

6. **Use earplugs and an eye mask**. These will help you to completely zone out and block out any distracting noises or lights. Some eye masks can also be weighted or cooling, giving you a less puffy look in the morning, so win, win!

7. **Wear some lingerie**. If you are suffering from changes to your libido or low self-esteem and want to feel sexier, purchasing some new lingerie can really help. No matter your age or size, your sexuality should be celebrated and looking in the mirror and seeing your natural body in all its glory, with a little bit of support and adornment can help you do just that. Your partner may not mind either!

8. **Wrap your hair**. Thinning hair from lowering estrogen levels can't be completely prevented without hormone replacement but the process can be slowed down by protecting your scalp and avoiding too much friction or pulling on the hair. Wrapping, braiding, or covering your hair with a satin or silk lined bonnet at night will do this as well as retain moisture in the strands and moisturized afro hair is strongest.

9. **Remove your makeup well**. Wash, cleanse, and tone your face every night can help avoid breakouts and a dull menopausal complexion. Gently remove your makeup, dirt, and grime with natural oils such as castor, olive, or sunflower oil to support the skin in its overnight regeneration and the renewal of new cells. Then wash the skin with lukewarm water, avoiding the use of loofahs or sponges as they can carry bacteria—your clean hands are just fine. Pat, rather than wipe, your face dry with a soft towel being cautious around the eyes and finish with a toner and moisturizer.

10. **Keep a journal**. Writing down how you've felt during the day can feel therapeutic. It will act as an outlet and can even make it easier for you to see solutions to any issues. You can also use it to reflect

on whether your symptoms are improving or worsening. It's not necessary to write too much, just a few sentences can help, but being open and honest is key to relieving any mental burdens. If you're worried about someone else reading it, hide it in a concealed spot or use a lockable diary.

Going On Vacation

Time away from your normal routine can be a blessing but can also feel disruptive if not managed well. In order to have a smooth trip and make the most of this down time, preparation is key.

1. **Pack more than one outfit per day**. Being away from home means that you won't have access to your entire wardrobe, so ensuring you have plenty of spare clothes (day and night) will make you feel confident if you end up suffering from hot flashes and night sweats. You also never know how you will feel emotionally or mentally when you decide to go out in the evening, for example, so bring a few options if you can, just in case you are no longer in the mood to wear that little black dress.

2. **Pack period products**. Even if you've not had a period for several months, it is my advice to bring

three or four panty liners, sanitary pads, or tampons, just in case. The menopausal body can be erratic and you don't want to be caught out! You may also want to pack some wipes too.

3. **Bring a fan or other small cooling gadgets**. Whether you are visiting sunnier climates or not, having a hand-held fan (manual or electric) can be a life saver. They will provide a welcome breeze in sticky climates or help dry the sweat from a random hot flash. There are also neck fans which are wireless and hands-free devices that sit around your neck and treat your face to a cool and constant breeze with no effort. They usually have different speed levels that you can adjust to get the relief you need. Hot flash patches are also handy as they are small and easy to take with you on vacation. They can be placed anywhere on the body to deliver a cooling sensation. Some are infused with hemp extract for a calming effect day or night.

4. **Bring a scented item or essential oils**. Something that smells like home or your favorite oil can help ease your anxiety around being away from familiarity. You can spray a towel, pillow, or item of clothing that you can sniff when you start to feel uneasy.

5. **Remember your medication**. If you are taking HRT, antidepressants or any other medication, it's important to bring them with you. You may be on a break from everyday life but unfortunately menopausal symptoms don't take vacations and you may start to struggle without any remedies. Going "cold turkey"–stopping suddenly–with HRT can cause some problems with studies showing that it can bring a return of menopause symptoms that are much worse than before, because the drop in estrogen will be sudden rather than gradual. It can also cause high blood pressure. Stopping antidepressants abruptly can have similar effects and you may suffer from withdrawal symptoms such as restlessness, unsteadiness, and stomach problems.

6. **Let your friends and family know where you are**. If you are taking a solo trip, it will be reassuring for both you and your family to know where you are staying. This is best practice whether you are menopausal or not but, in this case, it can be helpful if any of your symptoms become worse.

Chapter 6:
Family, Relationships, and the Menopausal Woman

In any relationship, whether platonic or romantic, there are times when your affinity may be tested. Menopause is such a time because it is not something that happens in isolation, no matter how lonely it may feel. It can affect family dynamics, put a strain on friendships, and make living with a partner feel stressful but honest and open communication can make it a much smoother ride.

Family

Menopause often happens at a time in life when we are juggling a lot of things at the same time and playing a lot of roles within the family. You may be doing your best to be a productive employee while being an attentive partner and a loving mother. As our parents get older, they may also require looking after too, which can all feel very overwhelming while trying to manage premenopausal or menopausal symptoms as well. This means that having the support of your immediate and extended family is so important during this time because they can often offer some respite and relief.

Older Generations

The older female members of your family will thankfully be able to relate to what you're going through. Although their experiences may not have been exactly the same, they will have a pretty good insight into what you may be finding challenging. In your parents' or grandparent's generation however, menopause was not spoken about or acknowledged as much as it is today. Society in the 1970s or 80s had an outdated view of women who were at this stage of life and there are very few medical texts about it because the female body was not considered worthy of studying after its fertile years. In 1966, menopause was even described as "a serious, painful, and often crippling disease" and an illness that needed to cured as quickly as possible, so that only your doctor knew about it. This made a lot of women feel ashamed or silenced and it pressured many into taking medication they were not entirely comfortable with. This means that even though older women in your family will be able to empathize, it may be difficult for you to have a conversation with them about how menopause is impacting your life and gain some advice or support.

Fortunately, my mother was open to giving me some advice, saying to take each day at a time and to understand that, even though my body feels crazy, these feelings will not last forever. However, if you feel as though you don't have such an open relationship with your mother, grandmothers, or aunts but you do really want to speak to them about menopause, my advice would be to show them how times have changed and that many people are now having open conversations about our bodies and the changes it goes through as we age. There are podcasts, TV and radio shows, forums, and social media platforms dedicated to this topic, so showing them these will help them to feel more comfortable talking to you about it and help you release the burden of secrecy.

Teenaged Children

Your younger children, if you have them, probably won't understand or want to know the details of menopause, but they probably will have picked up on some symptoms. They are surprisingly intuitive and may have noticed that you have a shorter temper than usual or are a bit hot and sticky more frequently. Teenagers, however, may be able to relate a little more as they would have gone through puberty and had raging and fluctuating hormones in a similar way. This can be a great way to lead into a conversation with both your female and male children about how you've been feeling and why they may notice changes in your emotional and/or physical state.

Ideally, you would have told your child something about menopause before your symptoms start. This would make the transition a lot smoother and make it easier for you to explain how you feel and are coping once it arrives. For example, imagine if you or your child's teachers had not told them about puberty or periods and one day it suddenly happened to them! Traumatic, right? So, telling them about menopause in advance will soften the surprise and they are less likely to worry about you. In the UK, menopause was actually added to the high school curriculum when education secretary Damian Hinds agreed that menopause is an important part of reproductive health and should be taught to children as part of sex and relationship lessons. This isn't the case in the USA, so if your symptoms are in full swing, having your own conversations is even more important so that it is normalized and respected.

So how do you start the conversation? Small. Nuggets of information are better than having a long and in-depth talk about the flashes and the aches and pains. You could instead link your menopausal symptoms to their experiences of puberty. For example, if or when they talk about their hormonal breakouts, you could tell them that you understand because you are also experiencing it, but because of menopause. Humor also goes a long way and may even help you see the funnier side of menopause too. For example, if your child buys some new tweezers for their eyebrows, you could ask them to borrow it for your chin instead! This may literally raise a few eyebrows and cause a little chuckle but more importantly, it can open up a relaxed conversation about the redistribution of hair that is caused by your hormones changing too. Also reassure them that any overwhelming and turbulent feelings you are both feeling are similar but temporary, and will return to stability once your hormones settle down. So ultimately, being informed, open, and empathetic to their own changes will in turn make your journey feel less lonely.

This is, of course, the ideal situation, but we all know that we don't always have the most patient and talkative teenagers. You are both going through such significant times of your lives which may cause clashes, so my advice in this instance would be to take your time, not downplay their feelings, and explain that you are struggling but working hard to feel and communicate better. Afterall, your children love you and don't want you to suffer, and by being transparent you will appeal to their better nature and they will most likely show some support and understanding. Failing that, there's nothing wrong with some alone time!

Alone Time

As much as we all love our family, some time away from them might be necessary. Don't feel guilty about this–your support network will understand. Feeling lonely is different from being alone, so although menopause can feel lonely at times, wanting some time to yourself is perfectly normal. You can use this time to unwind, pamper your aching muscles, and have a whole bed to yourself.

Being alone means that you can be selfish in the best way. You don't need to compromise your time or desires and be free to soothe yourself in ways you can't or feel awkward about when you are around family, for example, stripping down and walking around completely naked all day when you are experiencing a hot flash! Feel like staying in your pajamas all day and snacking on ice cream for a few hours without having to share? You can do it! This time by yourself will also allow you to get to know yourself and your symptoms better.

There are also scientific reasons why some time away from family will be beneficial, especially during menopause. It increases productivity and can help you build mental strength. When you are with your family, you can become distracted which can worsen your brain fog because people generally perform better when they have a little privacy. Being alone also gives you time to plan and make crucial decisions about your life, including your menopause treatment. As well as this, solitude sparks creativity, so you are more likely to find more personal solutions to your symptoms. So be proactive about making time for yourself. You deserve it!

Friends

Friends, especially girlfriends, can be the best support network during this time. Our friends are usually of a similar age, so they may even be able to relate to you more than you think. We generally also want to see each other thrive, so speaking to others about this time in our lives and what we need from them will usually be well received.

When going through menopausal symptoms, you may start to feel less outgoing in social situations than normal due to anxiety or depressive thoughts. Some women feel like they are no longer good company because they are less tolerant and find it more difficult to let go of little annoyances, even if they weren't bothered by them before. For example, if you tend to be the social organizer in your friendship circle, you may start to question why nobody else is making an effort to arrange dates or if you are the go-to "agony aunty", you may start to get frustrated that nobody is listening to your needs now. This is normal but sadly, it can make you slowly become more isolated. This sense of detachment often occurs because of our falling levels of oxytocin–love hormones–but it can be counterbalanced by talking into your feelings. Explain how you feel and re-address any boundaries that you think will be helpful while you are in this transition– these negative feelings will pass and your friends will understand. Being around friends can help with stress and anxiety around menopause, becasue you can use it as an opportunity to swap tips and advice or offload your frustrations and struggles. Start small by speaking to just one or two of your closest and most trustworthy friends at a time as I did, instead of messaging the entire WhatsApp group. This will feel less overwhelming and will avoid bombarding those who aren't as close to you with too much information at once. Don't be afraid to cry, laugh, and shout through your explanations because your honesty and vulnerability will be appreciated and help your friends understand the level of support you need. This is not the time to say "I'm fine" when you really aren't.

To help you feel comfortable enough to open up, you could alter the settings in which you meet up. For example, if you know that wine is a trigger for your hot flashes, and you usually meet in a bar, you could suggest meeting somewhere else, like a gallery or park. You could also meet closer to or at home, so that you have easy access to the comforts you need. When you have your catch up, it's important to remember that every woman's journey is different, so try not to compare your experience too closely to avoid anxiety.

If you want to make more friendship connections, you could try online apps, forums, or neighborhood hubs. This will open your circle without the pressure to show up when you don't want to. Online connections could be as superficial or meaningful as you'd like and offer a little escapism. You can have no filter and find out how other women outside of your demographic are working through menopause. You could learn something new while helping others out at the same time.

Being rational, honest, and reflective with your friendships can also help maintain your friendship among the rollercoaster of menopause. If you've been a bit snappy towards a friend, taking time to reflect on whether they deserved it or not and apologizing—if need be—can save a relationship. I even apologized before the irritation or snappiness happened and fortunately, they were great about it. True friends will get over it.

In the Black community, sisterhood is an unshakable bond that often keeps us going through all milestones and occasions in life. There is often an unspoken sense of joy and support when we see another Black woman win, whether we know her or not, and we will constantly remind each other of how fabulous and beautiful we are. For example, think back to that moment when Viola Davis won an Emmy and Taraji P Henson couldn't contain her excitement, giving her a hug and kiss as Davis approached the stage. Or when Toni-Amm Singh from Jamaica won Miss World and fellow Black contestant, Nyekachi Douglas (also known as Miss Nigeria), took the internet by storm when she ran around the stage in celebration for her sister in color. Miss Nigeria's reaction went viral with one person tweeting "when your friend starts a new business, podcast, therapy, anything that enhances her life, be her Miss Nigeria."

This support is also true when we are going through difficult times and we often band together and find ways to lift each other up, as authentically portrayed in the 2017 hit film, *Girls Trip*. So, stay close to your friends. You will need them and they will need you at some point too.

Romantic Relationships

If you are in a relationship with a Cisgender man, he probably doesn't understand the inner workings of a woman as much as you do, therefore, he may not be able to sympathize with your menopausal symptoms as much as you would like. This is why communication is so important.

Similarly, to your children, it would be best to talk to your partner about menopause and what comes with it before it starts happening to you, because speaking about it when you are already in pain, having mood swings, or are distracted can make it difficult to get your true feelings across. If you've already started having symptoms however, don't worry but be sure to devote time to having the conversation at a time when things are going particularly well in your relationship.

The key thing to remember during this conversation is honesty. Try your best not to lessen your feelings by saying things like "It's silly but..." or "I know it doesn't make sense" because this can make it seem as though your emotions are not valid. Instead describe how the symptoms you are experiencing make you feel in detail and why, and explain how you think they could affect your relationship. If you are in a mature relationship, these details shouldn't scare or put your partner off you because they embrace and love you for all that you are, and what you are going through is a fact of life–nobody's 'fault'. As someone living through menopause day after day, you are the expert and your brazen wisdom is more than enough qualification to speak about what you are going through without hesitation, judgment, or doubt. Also, the better your partner understands you, the higher your marital or relationship satisfaction. You will start to feel more like a team and may even find that they start to open up to you more as well. This builds trust and empathy during a time you both need it most.

If you can, speak to your partner about menopause face-to-face but if this is difficult or your schedules or living situation doesn't allow for this, a written letter can work well. Don't worry, your letter doesn't have to be beautifully and eloquently written. It could be a flow of consciousness, short sentences, or a list of words that describe your challenges, symptoms, and worries and you could read it out to them or give it to them to read alone. Once it's been read, it will be valuable to address and expand on anything that was mentioned so that you can see what your partner thinks about what you've said too. If your partner is a woman or is going through their own mental or physical challenges regardless of gender, you may find that there is some common ground based on their age. They too could be experiencing menopausal symptoms, anxiety, and body or self-esteem issues because this is quite common as we grow older anyway. This can make the discussion feel less daunting and the symptoms almost like a personal project you can work through together.

In some cases, your partner will listen but unfortunately not acknowledge the extent of what you are feeling. They may tell you to just relax or have a bath, and have a very simplistic view on how to 'cure' you which could be down to denial or having a lack of or false information about this time of life. This can cause ongoing disagreements and resentment can grow between you. If this happens, your instinct may be to just end the conversation and "agree to disagree" but this isn't the healthiest way to deal with it because you will end up harboring negative feelings for a long time and rot your relationship from the inside out. You don't know how long you will experience your symptoms for, so it's best not to brush it under the rug.

A great way to address this dismissal with a partner who is ignorant or naive about menopause, is to attend a doctor's appointment about it together. Your health care specialist will be able to give them the facts and sometimes, hearing the facts from a professional will make it seem more real to them. If you both want to continue the relationship, they will need to acknowledge that this is not just a "you" problem but rather something that needs working on together, otherwise it can feel extremely isolating and disruptive.

When it comes to sex and your changing libido, speaking to your partner candidly is especially important because making love and sexual intimacy is often the thing that distinguishes this relationship from your other relationships. Always say something if sex becomes uncomfortable or painful because if you don't, it can lead to vaginismus which is when the muscles in your vagina contract so much that penetration is impossible. It is an involuntary spasmodic reflex that your body does to protect itself and can disrupt your relationship and lead to frustration. To find it easier to relax, you may want to try talking about the sex-life you want and need. Exploring different ways to feel pleasure, trying different positions, and allowing more time to become aroused can also help but if these things don't work, it might be time to speak to a sex therapist. They will listen to your problems, assess whether the cause is psychological, physical, or a combination of the two, and aim to resolve them with medical treatment or certain exercises, such as pelvic floor contractions which strengthen the muscles involved in orgasm. Therapy can also help your partner become more empathetic and open to making changes.

There are also practical things that you can do with the support of your partner to help your sex life feel healthier and more satisfying during menopause. For example, if you or your partner smoke or drink alcohol, you should both consider giving up because both habits reduce blood flow to the sexual organs and can lower your estrogen levels further. Once you do overcome any issues around sex, having it more often can also help you have it more often! It keeps the tissues healthy and the oxytocin released will make you feel great, in and outside of the bedroom. But remember, just because you are experiencing menopausal symptoms, it doesn't mean that you are completely off the hook when it comes to pregnancy or sexually transmitted infections or diseases (STIs/STDs), so you should still continue with contraception until your doctor gives you the all clear if you don't want to get pregnant or pass on anything unwanted. The lower amount of lubrication in your vagina and the thinning of the vaginal walls during menopause actually make you more vulnerable to STIs. Ultimately, all of the people around us make us stronger. When we have a supportive network and relationships that have strong foundations, our hardships feel a lot easier to bear.

Chapter 7:
Menopause and Beyond

So, 12 months have passed and you've made it through the worst of the annoying, worrying, and disruptive menopausal symptoms. Your doctor has measured your follicle stimulating hormone (FSH) levels via a blood test and has said that you are now postmenopausal; Congratulations–I think! You get home from your appointment, sit down, and think "now what?" Some of us will feel an immense sense of relief that the worst is behind us but the rest of us may feel a little numb if those symptoms are all we've been feeling for a number of years. We've put so much effort into combating our nausea, hot flashes, and mental health struggles that, now that the effects have disappeared or dramatically decreased, we could end up feeling a little lost again. Both feelings (and all those in between) are completely normal and just require some time to adjust to.

Post menopause is when your hormone levels remain at a constant low, making your body function more predictably and your mind return to a relatively stable state. You will also no longer be able to become pregnant and won't experience a monthly menstrual cycle. But as a woman with low estrogen, there are things that you and your doctor will need to continue to keep an eye on, most of which are typical signs of aging.

Stay In Touch with Your Doctor

After menopause, you may notice that you are starting to regain your energy and not feeling as low or sensitive as you did before. But, although your symptoms may have subsided, you are still required to go for regular medical check-ups and screenings such as pelvic exams, Pap smears, breast examinations, and mammograms because these are all ways for your body to be monitored for any common issues found in postmenopausal bodies.

Pap smears, also known as Pap tests, are important to have approximately every three years at your doctor's discretion. It is a procedure that screens for the presence of precancerous or cancerous cells on your cervix–the opening of the uterus. It is usually a quick and painless procedure that is offered to all women aged 21 and over, during which cells from your cervix are gently scraped away and examined. You should continue to get these done whether you are sexually active or not and regardless of your age but women who have had a total hysterectomy for a non-cancerous condition and have no history of precancerous results may be able to stop having them once the reach menopause. You should always check with your healthcare provider before you stop attending your appointments as your lower levels of estrogen could lead to some abnormalities, so it's always best to make sure everything is continuing to be healthy down there.

Mammograms and breast examinations are effective ways to screen for breast cancer. During a mammogram, an x-ray image is taken of the breast tissue and usually involves two or more screenings of each breast. Whether you feel a lump or not, these images can help doctors detect abnormalities or cancer very early on which often leads to more successful treatment. Since mammograms can help with early detection, many insurance plans cover them but always check your specific policy. It is particularly important to continue with these screenings after the age of 50 or after menopause (whichever is the earliest) because unfortunately, the risk for breast cancer increases with age, with it being more prevalent in women who are over 50.

If you've never had a mammogram before, rest assured that it is nothing to worry about and usually takes less time than you think; around 30 minutes in total. The large machines may look intimidating to some but overcoming the nervousness may just save your life. There is not much you need to do to prepare for your appointment but most women find it more comfortable to wear a two-piece outfit on the day i.e., a shirt and pants, rather than a dress, as you will be required to undress from the waist up. It's also important not to wear deodorant, powder, lotion, or perfumes in this area because it can interfere with the results; showing up as small particles on the imagery. During the mammogram, the mammographer will place one breast onto a plate and another plate will compress your breast for less than a minute to help with the imaging. This will then be carried out on the other breast. It is normal for the compression to feel a little uncomfortable but always say if you feel pain. Once complete, your images will go to a radiologist who will interpret them and you will be contacted with your results within a week or two.

Your breasts are likely to have gone through a lot during your transition to menopause; from tenderness to becoming more lumpy to shrinking. This can make it more difficult to detect any problems with the naked eye, so it's always best to check them with a professional mammogram to make sure that nothing more sinister has developed too.

Another important reason to stay in touch with your healthcare provider is to check for osteoporosis. Losing bone is a normal part of the aging process, but in the first few years after menopause, women lose it more rapidly which can lead to weakened and fragile bones known as osteoporosis. It is not usually painful until a bone breaks but broken bones in the spine can cause long term pain. Postmenopausal women are more at risk of developing osteoporosis than men because the hormone estrogen, of which we have very little, is essential for healthy bones. This is why making sure that you are getting enough calcium and vitamin D is so important at this stage of life as they can naturally support the strengthening of your bones in the absence of hormones. If this is not enough to treat your level of bone vulnerability, then other medicines such as bisphosphonates, selective estrogen receptor modulators (SERMs), parathyroid hormones, or HRT may be prescribed.

Before menopause, women generally have a lower risk of being affected by cardiovascular disease, but post-menopause, the risk increases. Menopause itself does not cause it, but the lack of estrogen makes your cholesterol level more difficult to control, which increases the risk of fatty plaques building up inside the artery walls and this narrowing can lead to heart disease or stroke. Fortunately, keeping your heart healthy by keeping active, maintaining a healthy weight, avoiding smoking, and eating a healthy diet, can all help keep the risk of heart disease down, so I encourage you to speak to your healthcare provider, as well as friends and family, about gaining the support you need to achieve these lifestyle changes.

Finally, if you experience postmenopausal bleeding from the vagina, it is recommended to contact your doctor as soon as you can, even if it only happens once, there's only a small amount of blood, or you don't have any other symptoms. It is usually nothing serious but it can be a sign of cancer and cancer is easier to treat if detected early.

Some positive changes that may happen after menopause include the shrinking of uterine fibroids. Many women who are approaching 50 will develop fibroids which are usually benign tumors on the uterus. They are known to cause a lot of pain and bleeding and can press on the bladder causing discomfort and urgency. Fibroids tend to grow when estrogen levels are high, for example during pregnancy or at some stages of the perimenopause, so when estrogen levels decline post-menopause, they often shrink. This means that many women can avoid having surgery to remove them, so having menopause can give those who have them a much-deserved break from their symptoms. Other positives are that you stop losing iron every month through your period, so you are far less likely to become anemic, save money on sanitary products, and you can wear white trousers whenever you want to!

These indicators or suggestions are not here to scare you, but rather to protect you and keep you living a healthy and long life. Ignorance is not bliss when it goes to our precious bodies!

Maintain Holistic Health

As well as looking after our physical health, going through menopause should have taught us how important it is to take care of our mental, emotional, social, intellectual, and spiritual health too. We are multidimensional and complex beings and this doesn't change with age, in fact, we probably develop even more complex needs as we get older. With this in mind, many doctors and medical sites recommend following specific guidelines in order to maintain a healthy lifestyle when over 50, and it's as easy as remembering your ABCs... and D, E, and F. A is for avoiding smoke (including second-hand smoke), caffeine, alcohol, and excess salt and sugar. B is for consuming a balanced diet including whole grains, cold pressed oils, leafy vegetables, and nuts. This can relieve any hot flashes that you may continue to have after menopause. C is for calcium and D is for vitamin D, which both keep your bones strong. E is for exercise including weight bearing resistance training for at least 30 minutes per day. And finally, F is for food. Ensure that you choose foods that are low in saturated fat and cholesterol.

As well as this, OB/GYN, Dr Roz encourages her patients to follow a similar method to remember how to keep yourself healthy, but from a more holistic perspective and for postmenopausal women in particular. She calls it the "Dr Roz formula" for menopause and beyond and it is an acronym of her title and name.

D is for detox. Having gone through so much during perimenopause, it will be helpful to remove toxins from your body, both medically and spiritually. Cleanse your body by eating and drinking as cleanly as possible. To do this, it is recommended to drink at least 1.5 liters of plain water daily, eat regularly and calmly, cut out coffee and only drink a maximum of two cups of tea per day to help the adrenal glands. You can cleanse your soul by removing any negative energy around you. If you need to step away from certain friends, change career paths, or move house, then do it. It's never too late for a fresh start and you shouldn't feel guilty about doing this for the sake of your holistic health.

R is for rebalance. Addressing the balance of your hormones is often necessary through medical treatment but the balance of your life should also be addressed. Hormones do not cause cancer, despite it being a worry that has plagued women for years resulting in many of us suffering in silence. Instead, they are a means to a healthier and happier life, so Dr Roz encourages us to go to our doctors and seek the natural hormones we need. You should also aim to rebalance your life in general. A lot of time and energy has been spent trying to treat your symptoms and maintain the relationships that may have been affected during menopause, so now is a great opportunity for you to make your work, pleasure, family, and social time more balanced.

The next R is for resistance. Resisting sugar will be great for your holistic health as it can slow down the aging process, help you avoid problematic inflammation, stop mood swings, and reduce the chances of gaining excessive weight. Unfortunately, we can't eat the same way we did when we were 20 and expect the scales to read the same thing, so having a low-sugar diet should be considered post-menopause to avoid putting too much strain on our already weaker bones with excess fat. You should also try to take up some resistance training, as building muscle and performing movements that have slight impact will help make your bones stronger. The exercise will work wonders on your energy levels, mental health, and circulation too!

O is for oxygenation. Just breathe and enjoy life because tomorrow is promised to none of us. You should aim to do something that you enjoy every day and something that takes your breath away, in a positive way, at least once every month. For example, you could visit a beautiful garden or beach and soak in the breathtaking view or you could book tickets to see a performance or concert that makes you sigh with admiration and joy. Why not take part in yoga, meditation, or breathwork, or simply go for a brisk walk via a new route on your way home from work? Oxygen is the provider of life, the healer of cells, and a powerful weapon against stress, so use it wisely yet abundantly!

Z is for zoning out stress. Learning to say "no" and stepping away from drama is the best move you can make after menopause. In fact, it's a valuable lesson for all, as stress can induce a multitude of medical problems and it can even make your 'menopot' belly return or increase, so take control of your situation and make the moves you need to escape it. Listening to music is a great way to do this. For example, have you ever been in the middle of a stressful day at work or with the kids and then heard your favorite song play on the radio? If you have an affinity to music, it will almost instantly make you feel lighter and relieved as it helps you to mentally escape stressful triggers.

Using this, or the ABC formula, will help you start feeling more like yourself again, and ready to face the world head on.

Pass It On

Now that you've been there and got the menopause t-shirt, you could use this as an opportunity to pay your knowledge forward. Speaking to others about your experiences will help us as women heal and grow together as well as make society pay attention to our needs. You could share at events, contribute to podcasts, or, if public speaking isn't your thing, simply talk to members of your family, both male and female, about your experiences to help destigmatize menopause in the Black community in particular.

Your voice is so valuable, not only for Black individuals but also for scientific studies and statistics. If we don't tell medical professionals about our experiences and demand to be taken seriously, Black women's specific health concerns around menopause could go un-documented and therefore left untreated in years to come, which can leave us in the same position we are in now; underrepresented and with poorly managed symptoms. We need to be included in conversations about menopause and contribute to the discussions around the way we are treated because, after all, we are the ones it affects and I want future menopausal women to feel acknowledged.

Discussing our menopausal symptoms can also normalize them and make us feel less alienated when we reach this time of life. At the same time, it will make any symptoms that are out of the ordinary easier to flag and investigate more thoroughly, sometimes saving lives.

Enjoy Your Life

As the character Ryan Pierce said in the movie *Girls Trip*, "today is the last day that we will ever be this young" and with this in mind, I urge you to enjoy your post-menopausal life as fully as possible. In fact, 1950s anthropologist Margaret Mead found that many older women do just that and even get a rush of physical and psychological energy after menopause, due to energy no longer being used to fuel the hormonal cycle. Mead called this the "menopausal zest" and is quoted as saying, "there is no more creative force in the world than a menopausal woman with zest" (Busbee, 2022)! A survey for Health Plus magazine also found that 72% of women think they are "just as attractive" as before menopause, 82% feel "as feminine as before", and 8 out of 10 say that they now have an overwhelming "sense of freedom" (Independent, 2016). Furthermore, 6 out of 10 women said they feel better than ever before and feel an average of 10 years younger than their real age! So post-menopause is starting to look like something to look forward to rather than dread.

In 2020, Rhonda Burgess wrote an article for The Ethel e-newsletter from AARP, which was aimed at older women. She wrote about why we should celebrate the joys of menopause and in it, she says that she was determined to 'do' menopause and post-menopause differently. She stopped focusing on her perceived flaws and instead, looked at herself in a mirror naked and channeled her inner goddess! She was at the height of her newfound confidence and even found herself a new partner, so I urge you to use this time to take stock of your life too and look at it (and your body) with fresh eyes in order to enjoy a greater sense of self-assurance and empowerment.

With our modern care and technology improving both our health outcomes and longevity, we are living longer so we still have plenty of time to live our best lives after menopause. This time is to stop holding back, take the risks you need to, try new things, and taste as much of what life has to offer as possible. It has also been found that after menopause, your memory will return to what it once was, so build great ones that you can look back on fondly. Menopause is often referred to as "the change" so surrender to it and make it a positive change that is also as a beautiful rite of passage, because change can be good and we can't stop it from happening anyway!

Conclusion

The treatment and conversation around menopause is gradually changing and opening up. We've thankfully come a long way from the Victorians who didn't trust this time of life and said that it was making women insane. They would lock women up for "climacteric insanity" and attempt to cure them with a nice bath and a glass of sherry with dinner. In extreme cases, some doctors would use chloroform to knock women out or remove the ovaries with the hopes of making them more compliant, docile, and harder working! The 1930s weren't much better, as people described menopause as a deficiency disease and it was treated with testicular juice and crushed animal ovaries because the ovaries were seen as "the seat of feminine essence" (Singh et al., 2002). It wasn't until the mid-19th century that the middle-aged female body was taken more seriously in medical fields, and in the 1960s and 70s hormone replacement therapy was introduced and helped women feel liberated.

Fast-forward to today and I'm pleased to say it's no longer seen as the beginning of the end, but rather just the beginning. The beginning of a new chapter, the beginning of re-learning your body, and the beginning of new friendships and connections. Now, I am by no means downplaying the symptoms;

they are real, valid, and challenging and I can of course empathize with women who are finding it difficult but what if we think of menopause as a time where we get to pay more attention to our bodies and treat it more kindly than we've ever done. It's an opportunity to make self-care a priority and discover and reframe what it means to be a menopausal woman.

I hope that this book has empowered you enough to heal through your struggles, see the value in you as a woman, and to take advantage of the support that is out there that can help you to evolve into the woman you are becoming. You are a powerful woman and there are only two occasions in your life that you have no control over and those are when you are born and when you die. Almost everything in the middle is based on choice, so it's up to you to make the decisions that make your life as smooth, fruitful, and enjoyable as possible. You are your own agent for change and menopause doesn't affect that. You've raised your kids, you've supported your partners and, if you are alive and able to read this book, that means you have survived every difficult situation you've ever been through, so why can't you get through this.

I am firmly into my menopause and I can confirm that it can still be a great time to live life fully and I hope that my fellow sisters continue to talk about and destigmatize it.

References

Bakar, F. (2019, November 28). *The average woman spends around £5,000 on period products in a lifetime.* Metro.

https://metro.co.uk/2019/11/28/the-average-woman-spends-around-5000-on-period-products-in-a-lifetime-shows-study-11231543/

Behring, S. (2021, September 29). *What age do girls get their period?* Healthline.

https://www.healthline.com/health/womens-health/what-age-do-girls-get-their-period

Booker, L. (2016, February 5). *Which one is the mom? Photo goes viral.* CNN.

https://edition.cnn.com/2016/02/04/living/mom-twin-daughters-viral-photo-feat/index.html

Bryant, T. (2022, February). *10 biggest barriers to black mental health today*. Psycom.

https://www.psycom.net/black-mental-health-barriers

Button, K. (2021, May 13). *In our mothers' gardens: Reflections on black motherhood*. The Witness

https://thewitnessbcc.com/in-our-mothers-gardens-reflections-on-black-motherhood/

Catalyst. (2018). *Women of Color in the United States: Quick Take -Catalyst*. Catalyst.

https://www.catalyst.org/research/women-of-color-in-the-united-states/

Davis, R. (2020, October 7). *New study shows black women are among the Most educated group in the United States*. Essence.

https://www.essence.com/news/new-study-black-women-most-educated/

Devlin, R. (2019, November 29). *How to talk about menopause with teenagers*. Health & Her.

https://healthandher.com/hot-topics/how-to-talk-to-your-teenagers-about-perimenopause-and-menopause/

Elgaddal, N. (2021, November 17). *Complete symptom guide to Menopause aches and pains | stella*. Stella.

https://www.onstella.com/menopause-symptoms/menopause-and-aches-and-pains/

Ellery, L. (2014, July 8). *Hair and history: Why hair is important to women*. HuffPost.

https://www.huffpost.com/entry/hair-history-why-hair-is-_b_5567365

Femestella. (2022, February 5). *9 black celebrities on the importance of therapy*. Femestella.

https://www.femestella.com/9-black-celebrities-on-the-importanc-of-therapy/

Fenton, A. (2021). Weight, shape, and body composition changes at menopause. *Journal of Mid-Life Health, 12*(3), 187.

https://doi.org/10.4103/jmh.jmh_123_21

Gordon, D. (2021, July 13). *73% of women don't treat their menopause symptoms*. Forbes.

https://www.forbes.com/sites/debgordon/2021/07/13/73-of-women-dont-treat-their-menopause-symptoms-new-survey-shows/

Greaves, K. (2019, November 18). *"Life Is About Change": Black Women on Aging, Beauty, and the Power in Growing Older*. InStyle.

https://www.instyle.com/beauty/black-women-aging

Hicklin, T. (2018, January 23). *Factors contributing to higher incidence of diabetes for black americans*. National Institutes of Health (NIH).

https://www.nih.gov/news-events/nih-research-matters/factors-contributing-higher-incidence-diabetes-black-americans

Hill, A. (2020, September 30). *10 herbs and supplements for menopause.* Healthline.

https://www.healthline.com/nutrition/menopause-herbs

Holland, K. (2018, May 17). *Is hypnosis real? How it works and what the Science says.* Healthline.

https://www.healthline.com/health/is-hypnosis-real

Hostetter, M., & Klein, S. (2021, January 14). *Understanding and ameliorating medical mistrust among Black Americans.* The Commonwealth Fund.

https://www.commonwealthfund.org/publications/newsletter-article/2021/jan/medical-mistrust-among-black-americans

Jean, Y. (2020, March 11). *Black women have been using yoga for healing For decades.* Well and Good.

https://www.wellandgood.com/black-women-and-yoga-history/

Johnson, T. C. (2021, October 17). *Natural treatments for menopause symptoms.* WebMD.

https://www.webmd.com/menopause/guide/menopause-natural-treatments

Linshi, J. (2014, September 9). *9 ugly lessons about sex from Big Data.* Time.

https://time.com/3302251/9-ugly-truths-big-data-ok-cupid-book/

Menopausehealth center guide.(2022). WebMD.

https://www.webmd.com/menopause/guide/default.htm

Mental Health America. (2020). *Black and African American communities and mental health*. Mental Health America.

https://www.mhanational.org/issues/black-and-african-american-communities-and-mental-health

Oerman, A. (2017, August 31). *22 Period Facts That'll Blow Your Mind*. Cosmopolitan.

https://www.cosmopolitan.com/health-fitness/a12091987/period-facts/

Pacheco, D. (2020, November 6). *Can electronics affect quality sleep?* Sleep Foundation.

https://www.sleepfoundation.org/how-sleep-works/how-electronics-affect-sleep

Roth, E. (2016, December 8). *7 foods to help boost your sex life*. Healthline.

https://www.healthline.com/health/7-foods-enhance-your-sex-life

Singh, A., Kaur, S., & Walia, I. (2002). A historical perspective on menopause and menopausal age. *Bulletin of the Indian Institute of History of Medicine (Hyderabad), 32*(2), 121–135.

https://pubmed.ncbi.nlm.nih.gov/15981376/

TED. (2020). How menopause affects the brain [Video]. *YouTube.*

https://www.youtube.com/watch?v=JJZ8z_nTCZQ

TEDxTalks. (2017, December 11). *The woman you become with Rosalind Jackson.* YouTube.

https://www.youtube.com/watch?v=7rZp3JAPp_w

The 5 positive things you don't know about menopause. (2022, January 17). Busbee.

https://busbeestyle.com/5-positive-things-about-menopause/

Velez, A. (2014). *Menopause is different for women of color.* Endocrine Web. https://www.endocrineweb.com/

Ward, P. (2021, August 16). *What you may not know about African herbal and ecological traditions.* Healthline.

https://www.healthline.com/health/decolonizing-alternative-medicine-uplifting-black-agro-ecological-traditions

Why women feel great after the menopause. (2006, February 1). The Independent

https://www.independent.co.uk/life-style/health-and-families/health-news/why-women-feel-great-after-the-menopause-5544365.ht ml

Author's Note

Dear Reader,

Thank you for purchasing my book and taking the time to read through the material. I hope you received as much en-joyment from it as I did writing it.

I would like to take this time to humbly ask that you leave me an honest review on whatever platform you purchased this book from. I do take the time to read all of them to fur-ther assist me in my growth and to make improvements to my published works. This would be greatly appreciated, and I offer you my sincerest gratitude for taking the time to leave a review for me.

Most Gratefully Written, Tara.

Menopause and Me
Tara M. Iversen

© Copyright 2021 - All rights reserved.

…………..

The content contained within this book may not be reproduced, duplicated or transmitted without direct written permission from the author or the publisher.

Under no circumstances will any blame or legal responsibility be held against the publisher, or author, for any damages, reparation, or monetary loss due to the information contained within this book. Either directly or indirectly.

Legal Notice:

This book is copyright protected. This book is only for personal use. You cannot amend, distribute, sell, use, quote or paraphrase any part, or the content within this book, without the consent of the author or publisher.

Disclaimer Notice:

Please note the information contained within this document is for educational and entertainment purposes only. All effort has been executed to present accurate, up to date, and reliable, complete information. No warranties of any kind are declared or implied. Readers acknowledge that the author is not engaging in the rendering of legal, financial, medical or professional advice. The content within this book has been derived from various sources. Please consult a licensed professional before attempting any techniques outlined in this book.

By reading this document, the reader agrees that under no circumstances is the author responsible for any losses, direct or indirect, which are incurred as a result of the use of information contained within this document, including, but not limited to, — errors, omissions, or inaccuracies.

....

Thank you for buying this book.

www.ingramcontent.com/pod-product-compliance
Lightning Source LLC
Chambersburg PA
CBHW070948080526
44587CB00015B/2234